Praise for **The Family Guide to Getting Over OCD**

"Reading this book is basically like having Dr. Abramowitz as your family's therapist. There are many explanations and examples that helped us understand what our daughter was going through and connect with her in a healthier way. The real game changer was when we successfully stopped participating in her compulsions. Following this book's advice was not always easy, but it definitely improved our child's self-confidence and reduced the level of frustration in our family."
　　　　—*Len G., Wake Forest, North Carolina*

"If you have a family member suffering from OCD, this masterful book offers guidance and hope. Dr. Abramowitz helps you understand what your loved one is going through, what treatment entails, and how you can provide the best support. This is an impressive work that fills a significant gap in the field, and that will be helpful to everyone who cares about someone with OCD."
　　　　—*Eric Storch, PhD, Professor and Vice Chair of Psychology,*
　　　　　Menninger Department of Psychiatry and Behavioral Sciences,
　　　　　Baylor College of Medicine

"This excellent resource is packed with great examples. In simple, clear language, it describes specific strategies you can start using immediately to increase your support of your loved one—while reducing accommodation of OCD. This book is a 'must have' for anyone with an adult or child family member struggling with OCD."
　　　　—*Lisa W. Coyne, PhD, Department of Psychiatry, Harvard Medical*
　　　　　School; Director, New England Center for OCD and Anxiety

"By far the most comprehensive family-focused OCD resource. Dr. Abramowitz, one of the premier leaders in the field, includes everything a loved one needs to know in one easy-to-read book. He guides you through each step needed to help someone with OCD."
　　　　—*Bradley C. Riemann, PhD, Chief Clinical Officer,*
　　　　　Rogers Behavioral Health

The Family Guide to Getting Over OCD

Also from Jonathan S. Abramowitz

The Family Guide to Getting Over OCD

Reclaim Your Life and Help Your Loved One

JONATHAN S. ABRAMOWITZ, PhD

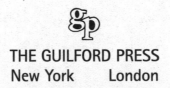

THE GUILFORD PRESS
New York   London

Copyright © 2021 The Guilford Press
A Division of Guilford Publications, Inc.
370 Seventh Avenue, Suite 1200, New York, NY 10001
www.guilford.com

Printed in the United States of America

Last digit is print number: 9   8   7   6   5   4   3   2   1

Library of Congress Cataloging-in-Publication Data is available from the publisher.

ISBN 978-1-4625-4136-2 (paperback) — ISBN 978-1-4625-4601-5 (hardcover)

To all the couples and families affected by OCD
who have shared with me their trials and triumphs

Contents

PART III

Reducing OCD's Influence Step by Step

PART IV

When Your Loved One Is Ready for Help

Purchasers of this book can download and print enlarged versions of the handouts at *www.guilford.com/abramowitz4-forms* for personal use or use with clients (see copyright page for details).

Author's Note

Families portrayed in the illustrations and examples in this book are composites of real people, thoroughly disguised to protect individuals' privacy.

In this book, I alternate between masculine and feminine pronouns when referring to a single individual. This choice was made to promote ease of reading as our language continues to evolve and not out of disrespect toward readers who identify with other personal pronouns. I sincerely hope that all will feel included.

Acknowledgments

First and foremost, I want to thank all of the couples and families I've worked with in my years of studying and treating people with OCD. They inspire me to continue working hard as a clinician and scientist to expand our knowledge and disseminate information through books like this one.

I also want to express my sincere gratitude to my most influential teachers—Kathy Harring, Joel Wade, Arthur Houts, Edna Foa, Marty Franklin, and Michael Kozak. Collectively, they taught me to appreciate psychology as a science and understand the often confusing signs and symptoms of OCD. I don't know where I'd be or what I'd be doing without their guidance and wisdom. Two of my current colleagues, Don Baucom and Lillian Reuman (who was a graduate student of mine), also deserve my thanks and recognition for teaching me about, and helping me think through, many of the concepts and strategies in this book.

Speaking of this book, it would certainly not be possible without the loyalty, enthusiasm, and wisdom of The Guilford Press's dynamic duo, Kitty Moore and Chris Benton, as well as Editorial Project Manager Anna Brackett. As my editors, they stuck with this project through thick and thin, guiding and encouraging me along the way. I am grateful for the way they got involved in the subject matter and helped me find my voice as the writer.

Last but not least, nobody has been more important to me during the time it took to write this book than the members of my family. I would like to thank my parents, whose love and guidance are with me in whatever I pursue. They are the ultimate role models. Most of all, however, I wish to thank my loving and supportive wife, Stacy, and our two wonderful daughters, Emily and Miriam, who provide unending inspiration.

Introduction

I'm sure you're reading this book because someone close to you has obsessive–compulsive disorder (OCD). You probably don't like seeing your husband, wife, or partner so anxious or your son or daughter spending so much time alone. Maybe you've caught your relative doing odd or excessive rituals or find yourself answering the same questions over and over. It could be that the joy and intimacy has been lost from your relationship. Or perhaps it's worse than that: daily arguments and power struggles, threats of violence and self-harm.

I don't have to explain how living with a loved one who has OCD can strain a relationship to the breaking point. You already understand that obsessions and compulsive rituals are relentless and demanding and cause the person you care about a lot of unhappiness. But perhaps now they are taking up more and more time for the whole family and you're tired of trying to convince your partner, child, parent, or sibling that the obsessions and fears are irrational and the compulsive rituals or avoidance strategies are excessive and unreasonable. It *seems* obvious that simple logic should fix all of this—which makes you even more frustrated when it doesn't. You've tried to resist giving in, but it only leads to more conflict and arguments.

Have things become worse and worse over time? Has your relative come to rely more and more on your assistance? Does she refuse to get help? Do you and others in your family disagree about how to handle the situation? Do you feel like you're at the mercy of your loved one's OCD?

I get it. I've worked with countless families affected by OCD. And I'm here to tell you that it doesn't have to be this way. You *can* turn things around. You don't have to walk on eggshells. You don't have to argue. You don't have to worry that "too much" anxiety will send your loved one "over the edge."

1

You don't have to arm wrestle him into getting treatment. The solution is to provide the kind of consistent support that helps your relative develop the confidence and skills to manage OCD in a healthier way and without needing to lean so much on you or others. Sure, it takes a good therapist and hard work to reduce OCD symptoms, but even if the person you love is reluctant to get help, there are things *you* can do to shrink the effects of OCD in your home, improve the environment, reduce conflicts and harsh feelings, and get family life back on track. Doesn't that sound nice?

If you're in a close relationship with someone who has OCD—a family member, intimate partner or spouse, or even a very close friend—I've written this book for you. It will help you understand what you're up against when a loved one has OCD. It will embolden you by correcting common misunderstandings and missteps that have probably gotten in the way when you've tried to address this situation in the past. It will teach you about the interpersonal dynamics that occur when a loved one has OCD and give you tools to help you avoid arguing and communicate more effectively. And it will help you take action to support the person you care about, breaking free of the vicious cycle in which your relative is trapped while *you're* working overtime. All of this will create more favorable conditions for your relative's recovery and for improvement in the home environment.

You might have read other books for family members of people with OCD, or perhaps visited a mental health professional to get advice for how to manage the situation. If so, you may have received some training in using cognitive-behavioral therapy (CBT) techniques, such as exposure and response prevention, to change your relative's thinking, behaving, and emotional patterns. But I'd be willing to bet you're reading this book because OCD is still a problem. As effective as these strategies can be, you can't force your son, daughter, spouse, partner, or parent to use them. That's why in this book we'll emphasize changing how *you* respond to your loved one's OCD. This focus will help you bypass the complications that stem from trying to control someone else. It's a balancing act—being understanding and empathic toward your loved one while gently, but firmly, refusing to participate in the OCD symptoms. And, of course, it will take patience and hard work. To achieve stability in your family and become the kind of support person your loved one needs, for example, you might need to set limits that the person with OCD may be unhappy with. That's why I'll also give you strategies for defusing arguments, managing your own stress, and moving from feeling desperate, hopeless, and guilty toward a much sturdier position of confidence and optimism.

The techniques you'll learn in this book have all been researched in clinical trials. It's a scientific fact that when this information and these strategies are used correctly, family life becomes less dictated by OCD, interpersonal relationships become more satisfying, and your loved one is likely to see a decrease in obsessions and compulsions—even if she chooses not to get professional help. And if your relative *does* decide to seek treatment, you'll have the skills to play an effective role and bolster its effects. Basically, I have taken state-of-the-art strategies that are proven to be useful in family and couple therapy for OCD and adapted them in a self-help format for you.

Who Am I?

I began working in the field of OCD as a graduate student in clinical psychology at the University of Memphis in the 1990s. Then, as a postdoctoral fellow at the University of Pennsylvania's Center for Treatment and Study of Anxiety, I had the remarkable opportunity to receive mentorship and supervision from some of the world's leading OCD therapists and researchers, including Drs. Edna Foa, Michael Kozak, and Martin Franklin. In 2000, I moved to the Mayo Clinic in Rochester, Minnesota, and opened the Mayo OCD and Anxiety Disorders Clinic—a treatment and research program of my own with a staff of dedicated psychiatrists and psychologists. People with OCD came to Mayo from across the United States and around the world, and I personally consulted with and treated hundreds of patients and trained and supervised numerous therapists wanting to learn how to help people with OCD. I also wrote and edited my first three OCD books (for professionals) while at Mayo, putting what I had learned though my research, training, and clinical work in print for others to benefit from.

But it wasn't until 2006, when I moved to the University of North Carolina at Chapel Hill (UNC), that I came to really appreciate how much (and in what ways) OCD affects (and is affected by) a person's relationship with family members or with an intimate partner. That was when I began collaborating with Dr. Donald Baucom, a colleague at UNC and an internationally recognized expert in the field of interpersonal relationships. Dr. Baucom and I received a grant from the International OCD Foundation (IOCDF) to develop and evaluate a treatment program for families affected by OCD. Our work together, which has continued to this day, has truly expanded my understanding of the interpersonal aspects of OCD and opened the door to many novel and fascinating research directions. But most important, it has taken my work as a clinician to a whole new level. Whereas I once felt that it was *sometimes* important to involve family members when treating a person with OCD, I now view this as *essential*. I consider OCD a "family affair," and as part of therapy I teach family members how to do their part to properly support their loved one while also keeping their family in balance.

Although this is not always an easy task, I love my work. I appreciate the stories I hear from people with OCD and their loved ones and welcome the challenge of understanding how each family and couple deals with obsessions and compulsions. Most rewarding to me is helping people like you learn and apply skills to help your loved one with OCD and reduce the demands of this disorder on families and significant others. Given my interest in and love of this work, and the extraordinary learning experiences I've been fortunate to have as a therapist and a researcher, writing a book for people whose relationships and families are affected by OCD seemed like the best thing I could do for all those I can't work with face to face.

How Can This Book Help You?

If there's one thing that's become clear to me through my work with patients and families, it's that people who live with a loved one who has OCD need skills and support every bit as much as the person with OCD needs treatment. It's not that you have problems of your own or that your loved one's OCD is somehow *your* fault—it isn't. But as you will learn in this book (if you haven't already figured it out from experience), trying to directly change your loved one's thoughts and behaviors doesn't work. In fact, it's likely to make your relative even *more* defensive, adding fuel to the OCD fire. So it's important for you to realize that only by becoming more familiar with the nature of OCD and by changing your *own* behavior (which you actually *can* control) will you be able to support your loved one in an effective way and avoid much of the frustration that comes from trying to arm-wrestle someone into feeling and acting differently. In addition, when you interact more successfully with your loved one and develop strategies for setting boundaries and freeing yourself from the need to argue or give in to OCD, you'll see your own—and your loved one's—morale and sense of competence improve. In turn, you'll experience a meaningful change in your attitude toward your loved one and in your relationship.

That's why this book, unlike others you'll find online or in your local bookstore, is going to make you an expert on OCD and how it affects individuals and families. Next, it's going to help you translate this knowledge into taking positive action to increase effective communication with your loved one, cut back on ways that you (perhaps without realizing it) might be enabling OCD symptoms, better manage your own frustration, and repair the harm that OCD may have caused in your family and relationships. I can't guarantee that this will be easy; in fact, some of the suggestions I make might seem challenging or counterintuitive. But try to remember that sometimes the solutions that seem most commonsensical are not the most likely to work (after all, one reason you've picked up this book is that other things you've tried haven't helped enough). So, please be open to new ideas and be willing to try things out.

On a related note, this is a self-help book—meaning it's designed for you to use on your own—but it's not intended to *replace* working with a qualified mental health practitioner should you or your entire family want or need professional help. You can use this book in any of these ways:

As a supplement to working with a therapist. Is your loved one getting treatment for OCD? Did your relative (or the person's therapist) recommend that you learn more about it? One of my reasons for writing this book is to have a good resource for the families of my own patients to use as their loved one progresses through treatment. If your loved one has tried therapy without much success, it may be that the therapist is not an OCD specialist. Or perhaps the clinician is just not accustomed to addressing OCD as it affects the family. If your loved one is already working with a professional he likes, you may want to share this book to help the clinician better understand what you are going through as a family and learn about tools for helping you manage better.

If your loved one is uncooperative or refuses to get help. It's the nature of OCD itself that leads many of its sufferers to resist help at first (as you'll learn in Chapter 5). But rest assured your loved one also wants to cope better, restore healthy relationships, and be happier and more independent. This book will help you more consistently align yourself with her own desire for happiness and independence. You may be surprised to find that your loved one becomes increasingly receptive to the kind of optimism and leadership I will teach you to use. What's more, these strategies are likely to begin nudging your relative toward getting the necessary professional help.

If you are looking for additional emotional support. The stories and examples you will read here—composites of real people and real situations I have observed—will help you see that you are not alone in your struggle to manage with a loved one who has OCD. The families I counsel often feel ashamed of the predicament they are in, *despite the fact that they are not to blame for OCD or the relationship dynamics that typically occur in families affected by this condition.* Shame and guilt, which are obstacles to improvement, get swept away the more you see how OCD comes uninvited into innocent people's lives.

If someone you love has OCD and it is affecting your family and relationships, but you never get to see a mental or behavioral health professional—much less a professional with the degree of training and experience needed to successfully navigate the thorny interpersonal aspects of this problem—I am pleased to have the opportunity to teach you about OCD and help you learn to provide the kind of healthy support that will start to turn things around. If you are using this book while also working with a therapist, I am delighted to lend a helping hand. If you are a therapist who doesn't have a lot of experience with OCD from an interpersonal perspective, I hope this book will be helpful in your work.

What's Inside?

This book is divided into four parts. Part I, which contains Chapters 1 through 4, will give you a foundation for understanding OCD, how it affects your loved one, and how it affects—and is affected by—family or relationship dynamics. You'll also learn about effective treatment for OCD, which is the basis for the strategies in this book. Next, the chapters in Part II (5, 6, and 7) will prepare you to take action by putting you in the proper mindset and giving you some tools for successful communication. Then, in Part III (Chapters 8–13), I'll walk you step by step through a program that will turn you into a more confident and competent support person for your loved one. You'll create a plan and tactfully notify your loved one, establish healthy limits and boundaries, and reduce your (and others') involvement in OCD symptoms while increasing your success in managing conflicts—if and when they arise. Finally, Chapters 14 and 15, which make up Part IV, will help you locate the right kind of professional help for your loved one (when she is ready) and then play a supporting role in treatment.

To help you get the most out of this book, I've included plenty of examples that illustrate the symptoms of OCD and the techniques I describe, along with some forms you can use to record and keep track of information as necessary. I've also carefully considered in what sequence the chapters appear so that each builds on the previous ones. For this reason, I recommend reading them in order. So let's begin! Chapter 1 launches your journey toward feeling more confident about your ability to support your loved one with OCD, more satisfied in your relationship with your relative, and more optimistic about family life.

PART I

Understanding OCD

1

What Is OCD?

I want to set the record straight right up front: OCD is a real psychologi-cal disorder that can torment and debilitate its sufferers, not to mention the upheaval and anguish it brings to people—like you—who love someone afflicted with this condition. It's not something your loved one is making up. Studies show that OCD affects 2–3% of adults and 1–2% of children. That's about one in every 40 to 50 people, not even counting millions more who experience obsessions and rituals that don't fully meet the diagnostic criteria. Research indicates that OCD is more common than bipolar disorder, eating disorders, and autism spectrum disorder.

Your relative didn't ask to have OCD. And given a choice, she'd opt to get rid of it in a heartbeat. Although she might not show it, she also regrets that OCD has placed a strain on your family. And even if she denies it's a problem, she'd prefer life to be better—for herself and for you. You see, OCD is like a very personalized form of torture . . . and no one likes being tortured.

There are lots of misconceptions about OCD, and if you don't actu-ally have the disorder, it's difficult to fully understand what the person you care about is going through. Not surprisingly, many people with OCD feel that their family members don't "get it." Maybe your ideas about OCD are influenced by the media. Countless movies, shows, and books have tried to portray OCD through characters such as Melvin Udall (played by Jack Nich-olson) in the movie *As Good as It Gets* and Adrian Monk (played by Tony Shalhoub) in the series *Monk*. Even in Shakespeare's literary classic *Macbeth*, Lady Macbeth compulsively washed her hands. And the list of celebrities with OCD seems to grow longer and longer each year, almost as if it's "in" to have this diagnosis. But the popular media often misrepresent this serious men-tal health condition. And you've no doubt heard people say that they're "so

OCD" about things like cleaning, organizing, or other personal quirks. But throwing around this term as if it's a cutesy nickname is disparaging to the people who suffer with the disorder. Is it any wonder OCD is so misunderstood?

My aim in this chapter is to give you an overview of what OCD is—the thoughts and feelings your relative is experiencing that you often can't see and the behaviors you *can* see and probably find baffling. In the next chapter I'll explain the underlying mechanisms that have trapped your loved one—and often end up entangling you as well.

OCD: Thoughts, Emotions, and Actions

The best way of thinking about OCD is as a collection of (1) unwanted private experiences and (2) behavior patterns aimed at trying to control these private experiences. As the box on the facing page shows, the private experiences are nonsensical thoughts, ideas, mental images, and doubts—called *obsessions*—that intrude into your loved one's mind even though he doesn't want them there. These obsessions, which are often triggered by something in the environment, provoke anxiety, fear, and uncertainty that something bad might happen or has already happened. To your loved one, obsessions are very upsetting and urgent, and they seem to require full attention and dedication; and yet no matter how hard he tries to get rid of these thoughts, they don't go away. Obsessions can be about virtually anything your loved one finds disturbing, but the most common themes tend to be the possibility of mistakes, bad luck, disasters, harm, and contamination. Obsessions that focus on upsetting thoughts about violence, sex, religion, and morality are also common. Along with anxiety-provoking thoughts, your loved one might notice physical changes, such as a racing heart, muscle tension, and an upset stomach—what's called the "fight-or-flight" response.

Now, imagine how you would feel if you couldn't get a fear-provoking thought that something awful was about to happen—or had already happened and was your fault—out of your mind. You would want to do whatever you could to prevent or protect yourself and others from the feared disaster. Your loved one, too, experiences a strong urge to reduce the fear, anxiety, and uncertainty associated with obsessions; after all, no one likes distressing thoughts and feelings. *Rituals* (sometimes called *compulsive rituals*) and *avoidance* strategies are the kinds of behavior patterns your relative uses to cope with obsessions, restore a sense of safety and certainty, and reduce anxious feelings. More or less any behavior can turn into an OCD ritual if it is

Components of OCD

Unwanted private experiences	Behaviors in response to the private experiences
• Obsessions—senseless, intrusive, unwanted thoughts, doubts, and images that keep recurring despite trying everything to get rid of them	• Compulsive rituals, "mini-rituals," mental rituals, avoidance
	• Provide short-term escape from the unwanted private experiences
• Anxiety, fear, and uncertainty provoked by obsessions	• Become ingrained habits that take up time and interfere with life
• Body sensations (racing heart, dizziness, etc.) caused by anxiety	• Family members often become pulled into "helping" with these behaviors

intended to lessen obsessional fear, yet the most common rituals are excessive washing and cleaning, checking, seeking reassurance, ordering and arranging, and repeating routine behaviors such as tapping the wall and walking through doorways. Some rituals also occur exclusively in your loved one's mind, such as excessive praying, analyzing situations, and thinking a "good" thought to replace a "bad" one.

There are two important points here:

1. *Obsessions are unwanted thoughts that provoke fear, uncertainty, and discomfort.*

2. *Compulsive rituals and avoidance are your loved one's attempts to reduce the distress associated with obsessional thoughts.*

Although rituals and avoidance sometimes succeed in controlling or reducing obsessions in the short term, they tend not to work over the long term; so your loved one finds himself doing more and more of the same rituals and avoidance behaviors. Over time, these patterns begin to occupy more and more space in the person's life. Perhaps significant parts of his day are taken up fighting obsessions and performing rituals. Perhaps this interferes with, or takes him away from, other important or valued activities such as homework, child care, a job, exercising, a vacation, intimacy, or just being in the moment. And quite possibly, what has brought you to this book is that these rituals are beginning to take up a big part of *your* life too.

What Is It Like to Have OCD?

What it's like to have OCD for one person can be very different from what it's like for another, as the following four individuals illustrate. Underlying their different symptoms, however, you'll undoubtedly begin to spot the obsessional and ritualistic patterns just described: recurring agonizing thoughts about an urgent problem that could be lurking and the need to address it and restore a sense of safety and certainty. We'll follow these four people throughout this book. Maybe you'll find similarities between their chronicles and what you and your relative with OCD go through. I'll use their (and others') stories as examples to show you how to implement the various skills and suggestions I present as you progress chapter by chapter.

Eduardo: "Everything Is Contaminated!"

"I was 12 when I started worrying about 'bathroom germs' and washing my hands forever after using the toilet. I was afraid I might get sick if I didn't get *all* the germs off. As the years passed, things got worse, and I started showering and changing my clothes every time I used the bathroom. I even started thinking that germs could spread to the sink, door knob, and other areas in my house, so I couldn't resist cleaning these things. I figured the rest of my family wasn't as careful about germs—I once saw my dad use the bathroom and not wash his hands—so I avoided touching anything that they had touched. Remote controls, chairs, computer keyboards, and doors were all off limits for me unless I made sure they had been cleaned thoroughly. Now I'm 17 and basically stuck in my room because I'm afraid my house is full of germs from my family, visitors, and things they bring inside—mail, groceries, their clothes, and germs from the hospital where my dad works. I have all kinds of washing and wiping routines, so it takes me about 2 hours to use the bathroom, take a shower, and get dressed every day. After my morning routine, I spend my day in my room doing schoolwork, playing video games, and chatting with my online friends. My mom stays home and homeschools me."

Ariel: Fires and Floods and Thieves (Oh My!)

"I'm 34, and I have obsessive thoughts all the time about making mistakes and causing disasters. *What if I didn't turn off the iron and it leads to a fire? What if I start a flood because I didn't turn off the water completely? What if someone breaks into our house and it's my fault that the door wasn't locked?* No matter what I do, I can't seem to get these awful ideas out of my head. So checking the appliances, electrical outlets, water faucets, and doors over and over is my way of making sure things are OK so I can calm down. The problem is that I'm often late, and it holds up the rest of the family (I have a husband and two young kids). For instance, there's a 20-minute checking routine I go through every time I leave the house. I have to check everything five times and count in my head as I'm doing it. Sometimes I write it down so I can check that I checked! At bedtime I have to know that the doors are locked and everything is safely turned off, so I check and then ask my husband to reassure me. I'm a teacher, and sometimes I get obsessional thoughts at work: *What if I hit someone with my car on the way to school but didn't realize it? What if I made a mistake grading a student's paper? What if I forgot to turn off the iron before leaving home?* I've even made up excuses so I can go home in the middle of the day to check that I turned everything off and locked up."

Xavier: Beyond Faith

"I'm 30 and live at home with my parents. I constantly obsess that I've accidentally offended God. *What if I didn't fully appreciate the food that He provides? What if I used His name in vain without realizing it? What if I didn't set a good moral example and I influenced someone else to commit a sin?* Because of this fear, I compulsively pray and ask God for forgiveness. The prayers have to be said perfectly and without any distractions; otherwise I have to repeat them until I feel God has heard them clearly. And I avoid using bad language, telling tasteless jokes, and attending movies that promote social liberalism. Drinking alcohol and having sex or masturbating are also off limits. I also spend hours each day reviewing my activities to make sure nothing could be misunderstood by God (or by other people) as improper or immoral. I usually end up asking my father for reassurance, for example, 'Dad, did I tell any dirty jokes to the kids in the neighborhood today?' Lately, I've been afraid that when I was a teenager I might have gotten my girlfriend pregnant. We never had sex, but one time I got an erection while I was kissing her. We were fully dressed, but I have this silly idea that she somehow became pregnant and then had an abortion. I often talk to my parents and pastor about this fear, and they tell me I have nothing to worry about. Still, I feel that I can't take any chances—I'm terrified I will end up in hell."

Linda: The Wrong Thoughts at the Worst Times

"I've had OCD since I was a young woman, but things got worse when my granddaughter, Emma, was born. Every time my son would bring the baby over to visit, I would get awful thoughts of inappropriately touching her genitals. I have tried distracting myself by thinking about anything else, but the horrible thoughts keep popping into my head. Am I secretly a pedophile? My husband (Nicholas) reassures me that I'm not, but I can't stand these thoughts. So, I've started avoiding the baby. She is no longer allowed in our house—Nicholas has to go to our son's home to visit her for both of us. We've also put away all the pictures of Emma that we'd displayed around the house because they trigger sexual thoughts. And things are getting worse. I have to avoid anything that's the least bit sexually suggestive, like some of our favorite TV shows such as *Dancing with the Stars* and *The Bachelor*. When the thoughts do come up, I find myself trying to figure out if I could really be attracted to a baby. Nicholas tells me he sometimes has bizarre sexual thoughts, too, and that it's just my mind playing tricks on me. But what kind of a grandmother has to avoid her granddaughter like this!?"

What Are Obsessions?

As noted above, obsessions are persistent unwanted thoughts, doubts, or images that your loved one finds strange and bizarre, that are at odds with her personality, beliefs, and morals, that she tries to ignore or dismiss (often unsuccessfully), and that make her feel very fearful, anxious, or guilty. Before you read about different types of obsessions, here's what obsessions are not:

- Extreme interest in a favorite song, video game, TV show, or even a potential romance.

- Worry, which is often a sign of generalized anxiety disorder (GAD). Worries concern real-life circumstances such as work and school, relationships, health, and finances (for example, "What if my elderly father has a stroke while I'm out of town?").

- Rumination, another form of repetitious negative thinking. Ruminations are signs of depression and involve repetitive thoughts about an actual problem or negative event (such as a poor grade or the loss of a job) that you can't seem to get past.

Types of Obsessions

Your loved one's obsessions likely fall into one or more broad categories, including the following:

Responsibility for harm and mistakes. Some people with OCD have intense anxiety and persistent thoughts that they've been careless and injured someone else, fearing that they will give their child the wrong dosage of a drug or, like Ariel, that a door was left unlocked, or an appliance or electrical outlet will start a fire. They may obsess about whether they've done enough to prevent such a disaster or believe that certain words (like *jinx*) or numbers (like 13) will cause bad luck or harm.

Contamination. Intense anxiety, disgust, or concerns with contamination from germs, bodily fluids or wastes (for example, blood, saliva, urine, or semen), dirt, animals, certain foods, or potentially harmful chemicals (for example, pesticides, fertilizers, and asbestos) are another common type of obsession. Maybe your fiancée is afraid to go to certain places or be around certain "contaminated" people, your partner is preoccupied with germs in bathrooms, or your sister worries about catching a sexually transmitted disease and then spreading it to others.

Order and symmetry. An excessive preoccupation with exactness, evenness, balance, and the need for things to be arranged "just right" might take shape as a fear of odd numbers or a need to have books or toys arranged in a certain manner. Some people fear that not arranging things in just the right way will cause bad luck (for example, if the picture is hung the wrong way, someone will die).

Violence and aggression. Those with OCD sometimes have obsessions that take the form of unwanted thoughts or images, or intense fears of physically harming people or animals they would never want to hurt—family members, pets, and even themselves. They might also have thoughts of hurting others *emotionally*, such as the fear of having insulted someone by using (or even thinking) racial slurs or other offensive or discriminatory behavior.

It's important to remember that these thoughts go against the person's typical nature—your loved one might be the most nonviolent or socially conscious person you know. Also keep in mind that these kinds of obsessions can be triggered by words associated with physical or emotional harm (for example, *murder, gun,* or insulting terms), stories about tragic events, or objects that could be used to commit violence.

Sex. Some obsessions focus on sexual preference or taboos and "perverted" topics related to sex, such as molesting children, incest, adultery, or sex with animals. Linda finds it awful and unacceptable to even *think about* molesting her granddaughter even though she isn't a pedophile. She worries that dwelling on such thoughts is a sign that something's wrong or that she'll do things she doesn't want to. Note that many people with these types of obsessions suffer them in silence because they often don't want to talk about these thoughts.

Religion and morality. Xavier has recurring thoughts that he's acted in sinful, unfaithful, or sacrilegious ways. Your relative might fear that he's sinned, falling out of favor with God, and will be punished; or feel excessively concerned with right and wrong and with making sure he's always acted morally. Professionals call these types of obsessions *scrupulosity*—which is a Latin word that means *seeing sin where there is none*.

Other types of obsessions. Your loved one might have other types of obsessions that don't quite fit into the categories just described. Maybe he has recurring fears that he's actually got a more serious problem than OCD, such as schizophrenia. Or he has intrusive, disturbing thoughts about a committed relationship he's in (for example, "Am I really, truly in love with my partner?"). Some people have obsessions in which unsolvable philosophical problems begin to cause a great deal of existential distress.

How Do People with OCD Deal with Obsessions?

To a person with OCD, obsessional thoughts seem like danger signals, and these danger signals drive him to engage in compulsive rituals and avoidance behaviors to restore a sense of safety as quickly as possible. In fact, those with OCD believe something awful will happen if they *don't* do these things. Therefore, they'll pursue these rituals and behaviors even if they seem unreasonable, take up loads of time, and cause rifts in the family.

Eduardo was afraid that if he didn't complete his cleaning rituals, he would get sick from germs in the bathroom. He avoided suspected sources of germs because he believed this kept him from becoming ill. Ariel's compulsive checking rituals were a way for her to quell her nagging fear that she was responsible for causing harm or disaster. Xavier avoided acting in ways he believed were unholy and repeated his prayer rituals over and over because of his obsessional fear that he might have committed a sin that would upset God. Linda felt that she had to engage in her rather extraordinary avoidance patterns to keep sexual thoughts about her granddaughter from coming to mind.

You probably recognize that such behaviors are unnecessary and illogical. But your relative views rituals and avoidance as absolutely necessary— the only way out of what seems like a frightening situation. This conflict is where OCD causes many problems with family relationships. You might keep trying to "talk sense" into your loved one, while he is convinced that performing rituals or avoiding feared situations is better than facing the threat of a feared outcome.

Types of Rituals

Like many people with OCD, your family member probably deploys different types of ritualistic strategies for dealing with obsessional fear.

Compulsive rituals. Those who get stuck repeating unnecessary behaviors over and over are probably engaging in compulsive rituals. These are often drawn-out and time-consuming routines and are likely the part of OCD that interferes most with daily life (both for your loved one and for the family). Compulsive rituals tend to fall into the following general categories: (1) excessive checking for safety, mistakes, or to make sure you haven't hurt anyone, (2) washing or cleaning to excess, (3) repeating routine actions such as rereading, counting, or touching, and (4) ordering and arranging things in a certain way. These are just classic examples—your family member may well have compulsive rituals that are not listed here.

Mini-rituals. Your family member might also perform mini-rituals— subtle or brief strategies for controlling anxiety or dealing with an obsessional thought—like these:

- To counteract obsessional thoughts that her medication will spill out of her purse and a child will think it's candy, eat it, and become very ill, your wife wraps her pill bottle in three zippered plastic bags.

- To avoid feared contamination from contact with door knobs, railings, and the like, your son quickly and subtly wipes his hands on his pants or shirt to "rub off the germs" after touching things.

- To distract himself whenever he experiences an obsessional thought of committing violence against the family dog, your father hums his favorite song.

Mini-rituals may not immediately be recognizable as part of OCD because they can be just about anything that's done in response to an obsessional fear.

Mental rituals. Your loved one might have rituals that she performs entirely in her mind. Xavier, for example, would repeat the phrase "God is good" 14 times to himself (14 was a lucky number for Xavier) whenever he had the obsessional thought *What if I love the devil more than I love God?* This mental ritual "canceled out" or "neutralized" the devil obsession. Long ago, I worked with a man with obsessional doubts that he had become so careless that he'd actually cheated on his wife—engaged in sex with other women—without realizing it. His elaborate mental ritual involved sitting down at the end of the day and reviewing all of his activities to reassure himself that he'd not been unfaithful. If he was interrupted during this process, which might last hours, or if he lost his train of thought, he would need to start over from waking up that morning.

Mental rituals are relatively common. And because they're *thoughts* as opposed to *outward behaviors,* your loved one might not even realize they're a symptom of OCD—clinicians don't always catch them either.

Reassurance-seeking rituals. In addition to his avoidance, washing, and cleaning, Eduardo compulsively sought out infectious disease experts online to ask about risks associated with various diseases. After her nightly checking rituals, Ariel would ask her husband for assurance that she had really turned off the stove and locked the front door. Sometimes she asked multiple times just to be *absolutely* sure and needed to hear him say specific words, like *Yes, I am absolutely sure that I saw you lock the door.* Your loved one has reassurance-seeking rituals as well if she bombards you (or others) with repeated questions about whether she is a good person, about the results of medical tests, or even about supernatural, existential, philosophical, or other sorts of questions that you really can't answer definitively (for example, *Do I have free will over my actions, or are they predetermined?*). She might also try to get reassurance by *confessing* obsessional thoughts to you. It can be extremely frustrating if you're getting repeatedly drawn into providing this kind of compulsive reassurance or listening to confessions—but rest assured that you're not alone. This is a very common ritual, and in later chapters you'll pick up some strategies for putting an end to it.

How OCD Takes Its Toll

Obsessive fears and compulsive rituals take their toll in different ways. If your relative is like many people with OCD, she also experiences bouts of depression (about half of people with OCD meet the criteria for a depressive disorder). She might feel embarrassed or ashamed of her obsessions and rituals, like something is "wrong with her," and try to hide these symptoms from others. She might experience intense feelings of sadness, worthlessness, or hopelessness about the future. Such a mindset may result from the severe interference in social, work, academic, and leisure functioning that OCD often causes. Although suicide is rare among people with OCD, your relative might have occasional thoughts that life is not worth living. Such ideas are, of course, not to be taken lightly.

Most likely, your loved one began showing signs of OCD before age 25. Many people develop the disorder in their late teens or early 20s, when they're becoming more independent and are faced with greater responsibilities (maybe you noticed from the preceding stories that responsibility often plays a role in OCD). But OCD can start at almost any time during childhood (usually not before age 4 or 5), in adolescence, and even throughout adulthood. It can also be hard to pinpoint exactly when OCD begins because the symptoms usually come on gradually, although there are instances of OCD starting abruptly in childhood, during pregnancy, after childbirth, or after experiencing certain types of illnesses or a life-changing traumatic event. If your relative with OCD is an adult, he may have been dealing with this torment for a very long time. The good news is that treatments for OCD—including the skills you'll learn in this book for supporting your loved one—are very effective, and they don't rely on knowing when (or how) OCD started.

How Did This Happen?

Obviously no one would ask for OCD. So why do some people end up with it? Your loved one's obsessions and rituals are the result of a complex combination of biological, learning, and circumstantial mechanisms; and unfortunately, at this point we simply don't know enough about these factors or how they combine to give rise to OCD. So don't get sidetracked by the search for a cause. The strategies you'll learn to apply in this book for supporting your loved one require a keen understanding of how the symptoms of OCD work, but not their cause. And we understand these symptoms particularly well. Still, here's what we do know about possible causes:

Theories about OCD being caused by "imbalances" of neurotransmitters in the brain, problems with brain structure and function, strep infections, and genetics have all been raised, yet none has proven definitive. It also seems logical that OCD tendencies might be learned. Eduardo, for example, might have learned to fear germs from growing up in a home where he was often told that "germs are everywhere." Your loved one's problems with OCD might also have started following a trauma or abusive situation that made him think twice about his own safety and security. Another possibility is that experiences during his formative years led to an excessive sense of personal responsibility. When Ariel was 13, her mother became seriously ill for several months, and Ariel had to singlehandedly care for her baby brother, as her father spent much of his time working outside the home. It is possible that Ariel learned her need for certainty and checking behavior through these sorts of experiences. Similarly, Xavier's religious school teachers were very stern and would repeatedly warn Xavier that severe punishment awaited him if he didn't act morally, especially toward God. Xavier grew up worried that he wasn't obeying God's laws closely enough and developed his compulsive praying and reviewing rituals to try to ensure he was destined for heaven as opposed to hell. Finally, there might have been coincidences where it *seemed* to your family member that her thoughts or behaviors led to a negative event, causing her to become afraid of thinking negative thoughts. As with biology, however, the environmental explanations for OCD have not been proven as fact. In other words, we can't pin the cause of OCD on any one of these factors. In fact, many people with OCD say they've *never* experienced the situations just described; and there are loads of people who *have* had these experiences but never develop OCD.

The question I hear most often from family members of those with OCD is, however, "Did *I* cause my relative's OCD?" It's easy to fall into this trap:

- "He's my son, so I must have given him bad genes."
- "I raised my daughter, so I must have screwed up as a parent."
- "If I'd only stopped reassuring my husband, this problem would have gone away long ago."

As you've learned, OCD results from a complex set of factors that we don't understand very well. So your child's OCD is not your fault. Period. You're not responsible for anyone's biological makeup, nor did you deliberately arrange for any unfortunate experiences to occur. In a similar vein, OCD is not your relative's fault either—although many people with OCD look at the pain and suffering they cause their families and blame themselves. There's just no single person, event, or biological factor that can cause a complex problem like OCD. Playing the blame game not only leads to undeserved guilt and shame, but it will weaken your ability to provide the kind of support your family member needs. So, the question isn't "Did I cause the OCD?" but rather "What can I do to support recovery?" Just because OCD isn't anyone's fault doesn't mean that you and your loved one can't do anything to help the situation.

2

How Does OCD Set Its Trap?

OCD is like a professional scam artist. Scam artists survive by taking advantage of people's weaknesses, deceiving them into thinking they're getting a great deal or some easy money. But in the end, it's the scam artist who walks away with your money. Similarly, OCD tricks your relative into thinking that avoidance and rituals are the answer to obsessions and anxiety. When obsessions about germs show up and provoke the fear of contamination, just wash, clean, and avoid anything that could be contaminated. When obsessional doubts show up and provoke the fear of harm or mistakes, just recheck or ask for reassurance. For a moment, your relative might feel some relief from the obsessions and anxiety. But they always return. That's the scam.

Like any rigged game, this one can't be won by playing by the scam artist's rules. Your relative might invest more and more checking, washing, and other rituals into ridding herself of her fears, she might recruit you and others into helping, and yet the fears return—usually stronger than ever, forcing her to work even harder at the rituals. It's in our nature to try to solve our problems. So your loved one tries ever harder to figure out and fix the problem of obsessive fears. But OCD is not like the kinds of practical problems we solve every day. The harder she tries to figure out, control, or fight obsessional thoughts and fears, the more intense and scary they become—which leads to fighting even harder. Before long, OCD has your loved one—and probably *you*—deeply entangled in a vicious cycle.

That's not to say OCD isn't vulnerable. The key is to change the rules of the game.

Obsessional Fears: Same Situations, Different Responses

Have you ever noticed that you and your loved one with OCD might find yourselves in similar situations, but whereas you manage just fine, your loved one gets stuck with obsessions and rituals? Psychologists Aaron Beck and Albert Ellis advanced the idea that it's the way we *think about* or *interpret* events and situations—not events and situations themselves—that determines our emotions, behaviors, and even how the body responds physiologically. And it's certain types of interpretations that lead to certain feelings and emotions. Very negative beliefs about your self-worth ("I am useless and unlovable") lead to feeling depressed. If you view yourself as not living up to high enough standards ("I should have been nicer to my teachers"), you'll feel guilty. Similarly, when your loved one interprets a situation as threatening ("Driving on the 13th day of the month is dangerous because it's a bad luck day"), it leads to feelings of anxiety and fear, avoidance or ritualistic behavior, and perhaps muscle tension and a pounding heart.

Eduardo's mother couldn't understand Eduardo's fears of contamination. After all, when she used the bathroom she might think about germs but could say to herself, "Bathrooms are generally safe. The risk of getting sick is pretty low." But when Eduardo uses the bathroom, he tells himself something different: "Bathrooms are dangerous because they're swarming with germs that will make me very sick."

Eduardo's mother is able to use the bathroom, quickly wash her hands, and then move on to whatever else she has to do because she sees the bathroom as safe. Eduardo, on the other hand, sees the bathroom as dangerous. So his anxiety level rises, and obsessional thoughts about germs and illnesses race through his mind. He tries to control the anxiety and intrusive thoughts with washing rituals and avoidance, but remember that the game is rigged. Instead of being able to move on, he gets stuck. More thoughts: *What if I didn't get all the germs off? Should I wash up to my elbows? What if the germs spread to other places?* More rituals. More avoidance. The more rituals and avoidance he does, the less safe he feels. Eventually, he's avoiding contact with much of the outside world, holing up in his bedroom—a sanctuary from the fear of contamination. The way Eduardo thinks about bathrooms is what leads to obsessional fear.

A "situation" that triggers a ritual can also be a *thought*. Whether we realize it or not, we're constantly thinking about our own thinking—making interpretations of the thoughts, ideas, and images that run through our mind. When Linda had obsessional thoughts about her granddaughter, she took them very seriously, seeing them as personally meaningful and threatening. She told herself, "Something's terribly wrong. A grandmother can't have these kinds of thoughts—not about her grandchild! What if I'm actually a pedophile? This is unacceptable. I need to make sure I never think like this." Linda's husband, Nicholas, sometimes experienced bizarre sexual thoughts going through his mind too (as we *all* sometimes do), but when they did he would say to himself, "My mind's just playing tricks on me again."

Linda became absorbed in the thought's *content,* rather than seeing the thought as just nonsensical. And the more she fought, avoided, and sought reassurance, the more she had the exact thought she found so unacceptable— and this made it snowball into a full-blown obsession. That's how she got stuck in the OCD loop.

Common Misinterpretations in OCD

Research shows that there are certain patterns of mistaken beliefs and misinterpretations that keep those with OCD perceiving situations and thoughts as dangerous, leading to obsessional fear.

Exaggerating threat. Eduardo overestimated the dangerousness of "bathroom germs," and Ariel overestimated the probability of fires, floods, and break-ins. If your loved one overestimates threat, then even senseless thoughts and ideas about feared outcomes will seem all the more real, leading to anxiety, avoidance, and rituals.

Assuming sole responsibility. When Ariel's intrusive thoughts about disasters, injuries, or deaths came to mind, she responded with the belief that she was wholly responsible for preventing such catastrophes or reassuring herself that they hadn't already occurred. If your relative feels he is solely responsible for disastrous events, he may get trapped by OCD in compulsive checking, reassurance seeking, and confessing (or warning others of potential harm). Ariel, for example, had time-consuming checking rituals and often asked her husband to reassure her that everything was OK.

Exaggerating the significance of thoughts. Does your relative with OCD take senseless intrusive thoughts that run counter to her usual personality and assume that they reveal some deep-seated evil, dirty, perverted, or immoral side of her? That's exactly what Linda did with her unwanted thoughts about molesting her granddaughter. Interpreting thoughts in this way can cause a great deal of anxiety and fear. Yet it's also incorrect: your relative's intrusive obsessional thoughts almost certainly mean nothing important at all. Still, this pattern provokes urges to perform rituals to dismiss or "neutralize" unwanted thoughts and reduce obsessional fear.

Confusing thoughts with actions. Sometimes people with OCD believe that (1) *thinking about* a negative event makes that event more likely to happen and (2) *thinking* of doing something bad is the moral equivalent of actually *doing* it (or wanting it to happen). Xavier feared that his senseless thoughts of acting immorally and being punished by God would come true. Linda felt that merely thinking (unwanted) sexual thoughts about Emma was as disgraceful as engaging in sexual behavior. Like judging thoughts as overly important, confusing thoughts and actions leads your loved one to wrongly see herself as mad, bad, or dangerous. You can see how such beliefs lead to anxiety and urges to do rituals to "put things right" or dismiss the unwanted thoughts.

Needing to control thoughts. Xavier also believed it was important not to think about topics he felt were immoral, such as sex and blasphemy. He assumed that to maintain control over himself he needed not to have any inappropriate thoughts. Even the *thought* of a racial slur or dirty joke seemed unacceptable. Does your relative believe that he can and should be able to control or dismiss his unwanted or upsetting thoughts or that he would be a better person if he could just exercise enough willpower to control his mind?

Having difficulty tolerating uncertainty. Chances are your relative feels he's got to have a 100% guarantee of safety when it comes to his obsessional fears. The trouble is, most obsessions focus on matters where it's hard to ever have ironclad assurances. This reality increases uncertainty and fear and may lead to excessive measures to try to resolve the doubt. Eduardo can't see germs, so he avoids touching things or washes and cleans to excess so he feels assured of being germ-free. Linda has obsessional doubts about who she "really is" or whether she'll do something awful in the future, which is unknowable, so the intolerance of uncertainty provokes in her overwhelming fear and urges to avoid and seek reassurance.

Obsessions Hit Your Loved One Where It Hurts the Most

Just like a scam artist, OCD focuses obsessional thoughts and fears on what a person values most in life. Think about the things your family member loves most or considers extremely important—maybe it's health and safety, caring for others, virtue, morality, sincerity, cleanliness, or religious faith. If the person you care about values being cautious and caring for others, her obsessions probably focus on the fear of making mistakes or being responsible for harm. If she prides herself on cleanliness and good health, the obsessions might pertain to germs, contamination, and the possibility of illness. Obsessions about violence and aggression are often found among the most sensitive, caring, and gentle people. Obsessions about sin and sacrilege mostly occur in people who take religion and their relationship with God very seriously. Obsessions that involve unwanted sexual intrusions are often found in people who consider themselves highly moral or whose sexuality plays an important role in how they view themselves overall.

Why Don't Obsessional Fears Reveal Themselves as the Scam That They Are?

The situations that trigger OCD fears aren't really dangerous, and the unwanted thoughts that have turned into obsessions are nothing more than harmless mental intrusions. Yet your relative continues to see them as signs of danger, becoming extremely fearful and wasting time and energy with rituals and avoidance. But if her obsessional fears rarely (if ever) come true, why doesn't she realize this and get over her fear? Why does she continue the disruptive behavior? The answer is that it's her rituals and avoidance—the very things she's doing to try to feel safer—that prevent her from realizing that her obsessional fears are irrational. Let's look more closely at how this works.

How Do Rituals Make OCD Stronger?

First, rituals technically "work" because they often cause an immediate reduction in anxiety. But even if it's only a slight or temporary reduction, the brain registers rituals as something to be repeated whenever a similar anxiety-provoking situation or thought shows up. That is, your relative learns to repeat rituals because they reduce her distress. What's more, each time this happens, the urge to do rituals gets stronger and stronger. In some ways, rituals might seem "addicting," and your loved one might even lie or make up false excuses for his rituals to protect his ability to do them (although we don't technically classify OCD as an addiction). Meanwhile, rituals gradually take up increasing time and energy, often reaching the point where they severely disrupt day-to-day life and get in the way of activities—both important and routine. To make matters even worse, the more rituals your family member performs, the more she is reminded of her obsessional fears, so more and more situations and thoughts provoke urges to ritualize . . . and the vicious cycle goes on and on.

A second problem with rituals is that they prevent your family member from realizing that obsessions *don't* actually signal danger. Let's say your son is afraid that the number 6 will cause bad luck, so he performs compulsive rituals—knocking on wood and saying a prayer—every time he encounters this number. As long as he does these rituals, he never has a chance to learn that the number 6 is actually safe. That's because when there's no bad luck, he'll attribute this to his ritualizing and continue to believe that he narrowly escaped disaster ("If I hadn't ritualized, the number 6 would have caused something awful"). Since he never really puts his fears to the test by *consistently* not ritualizing, the number 6 remains frightening and he continues to have urges to ritualize.

Perhaps the person you love with OCD has mistaken beliefs about experiencing fear, uncertainty, and obsessional thoughts. Your husband believes, "I can't function if thoughts about pedophilia are stuck in my head." Your wife tells herself, "I can't handle not being sure whether I'm going to heaven or hell." Your daughter thinks, "If I don't do anything about anxiety, it will go on forever, spiral out of control, and I'll lose my mind." Using rituals prevents your loved one from realizing that fear, uncertainty, and obsessional thoughts are also safe. That is, constantly using rituals to control or remove obsessions and anxiety prevents one from learning that these experiences, although unpleasant, are temporary and more manageable than they seem. And don't fall into the trap of thinking that just because mini-rituals and mental rituals are quick or subtle they're any less important than more time-consuming compulsive rituals. The fact is that anything your loved one is doing in response to senseless obsessional thoughts has a way of playing into OCD's hands and keeping the vicious cycle going.

How Does Avoidance Make OCD Stronger?

Avoidance also seems like a logical problem-solving strategy for obsessional fear. Anyone who fears that dangerous germs are lurking in public bathrooms would avoid such bathrooms. Likewise, if you believe that *thinking about* killing people is the moral equivalent of actually committing murder, it makes sense that you would avoid movies and shows with violence that might provoke such thoughts. It's just that these fears are based on mistaken patterns of thinking. Your relative is overestimating the danger associated with situations and obsessional thoughts. But, as with rituals, avoidance plays into the vicious cycle of OCD. Here's how:

For one thing, avoiding a feared situation and successfully steering clear of obsessional thoughts and anxiety (even if temporarily) leads you to believe the avoidance is effective, and so the pattern gets stronger. As a result, avoidance patterns tend to expand over time. Maybe it's manageable at first—only a few situations or stimuli are avoided; but in time, this grows so that life becomes more and more restricted.

Eduardo, who ended up confined to his bedroom, is a perfect example. He started out avoiding touching certain parts of bathrooms. But before long he found himself extending the avoidance to other places, eventually trapping him in a single room. As he began to fear new situations and places, he called up his avoidance strategy again and again because it seemed to work elsewhere. Such avoidance patterns may seem effective in controlling obsessional fear; but this only works temporarily. In the long term, avoidance further feeds into the vicious cycle of OCD.

Another problem with avoidance is that, like rituals, it robs your loved one of the opportunity to find out that feared situations or objects—and even the experience of obsessional thoughts and anxiety—are not really dangerous. If your partner, for example, avoids all shows or movies about serial killers, she'll never have a chance to find out that (1) these won't turn her into a murderer and (2) it's perfectly harmless to think about serial killers (think of police detectives, forensic psychologists, lawyers, and even actors playing certain roles, who spend their days thinking about and studying serial killers). Similarly, if you avoid public bathrooms at all costs, there's no way to learn that they are generally safe. To put this another way, avoidance keeps your family member from learning to correct the mistaken interpretations and other faulty thinking that leads to obsessional fear. This not only keeps obsessional fears alive, it allows them to flourish and expand.

Why Is Anxiety So Hard to Ignore?

The main purpose of rituals and avoidance is to control and reduce anxiety. But why can't your relative just put up with feeling anxious for a while until it subsides on its own? It turns out that anxiety works in a way that makes it impossible to ignore—and this is also part of the OCD trap.

Think about what happens when you feel anxious: your heart races, it's hard to catch your breath, you break out in a cold sweat, and anxious thoughts go racing through your mind.

When your relative with OCD becomes anxious, it's no different. These and other intense and unpleasant sensations seem to take over the body. This is called the *fight-or-flight response* because its purpose is to protect you from danger by preparing the body to fight back or run for your life. Eons ago, when humans lived in the wild with predators that were stronger and faster, having an automatic response take over when danger was perceived—for instance, an approaching saber-toothed tiger—was critical to self-preservation. Today, most of us don't need the fight-or-flight response to survive, but it's still there in the most primitive part of our brain just in case. And when your loved one experiences an obsession and perceives a dire threat, it triggers this built-in alarm response, resulting in an irresistible urge to escape from the anxiety.

Although everyone experiences anxiety and fear from time to time, people with OCD experience it particularly *often* and especially *intensely*. But even when it's intense or long-lasting, your loved one's anxiety response is not harmful or dangerous (remember, its purpose is to *protect* the body from harm). In fact, it's working in exactly the way it's designed to work. It's just being triggered at the wrong times, like when the smoke detector in your home sometimes goes off when you're cooking. The smoke detector is doing what it's supposed to do, but it's giving you a false alarm. And remember, people with OCD tend to overestimate risk and threat. So to your loved one, there are more and more situations and unwanted thoughts that seem potentially dangerous and therefore trigger these types of false alarms, which in turn lead to seeking safety through rituals and avoidance.

Putting It All Together: The Vicious Cycle of OCD

OCD cons your loved one into thinking something is dreadfully wrong and that there are strict conditions that must be met to resolve the problem and restore a sense of safety. Situations must be avoided and rituals must be done.

The diagram on page 30 shows how the person you love is ensnared in this self-perpetuating vicious cycle. The cycle begins with unwanted (intrusive) negative thoughts that may be triggered by something in the environment or that just come to your relative's mind without an obvious trigger. But misinterpreting these situations and thoughts as very threatening leads to preoccupations that provoke anxiety and uncertainty (obsessional fear) over the possibility that something is (or will go) dreadfully wrong. To cope with the obsessional anxiety, your relative turns to rituals and avoidance strategies that seem like they'd be effective ways of managing the perceived threat. But they're not. Rituals and avoidance might temporarily reduce anxiety or obsessions, but this tricks your loved one into doing more and more of them.

The Vicious Cycle of OCD

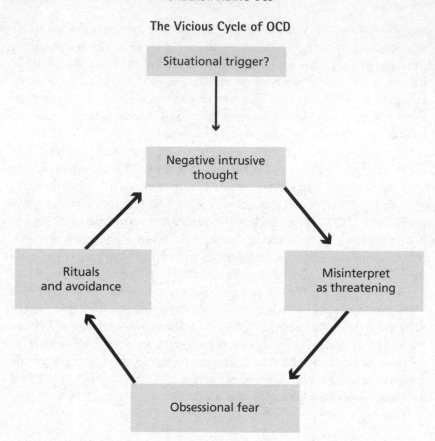

In the long run, rituals and avoidance keep your family member from learning that the situations and thoughts and the experience of anxiety are not as threatening as he thinks. So, the obsessional fear continues. As if that's not enough, over time rituals and avoidance end up taking up more and more time, energy, and resources—not to mention their negative effects on family functioning and relationships.

Now you have a good idea of how OCD is making the rules and setting a trap for the person you love. Chances are, though, that you're caught in the trap too. Understanding how you've become ensnared is key to getting untangled, preserving family relationships, and perhaps even helping your relative write new rules and get free of the scam of OCD. So, we'll turn to this in Chapter 3.

3

How Do Families Get Entangled in OCD?

You've undoubtedly picked up this book because in one way or another, your loved one's difficulties with OCD are affecting you and others in your household. This is a common occurrence for couples or families in which someone has OCD, and psychologists understand it well. Remember that for the person with OCD, the environment is full of triggers that prompt fear and distressing obsessional thoughts about seemingly dire and pressing threats. Your relative urgently turns to avoidance and rituals to reduce the apparent risk. It's his struggle to control the environment to maximize perceived safety and certainty that imposes on you or others in your family and sows the seeds for getting pulled into the vicious cycle of OCD.

How does this happen? Why do you and others get pulled in? For one thing, it's difficult to see someone you love in so much distress. So it's only natural to do what's necessary to protect her from these feelings or to try to talk her out of feeling afraid. But you've probably noticed that even if this helps quell distress in the short term, the strategies you've tried don't work very well in the long run. Your loved one eventually starts obsessing again and is once more compelled to avoid, use rituals, and ask for reassurance. Your loved one's apparent inability to respond to logic can be frustrating, leading to arguments. Such conflicts compound the distress and dissatisfaction in your family, which further exacerbates your loved one's OCD symptoms.

I've conducted studies on these patterns in couples and families, and I've seen how they unfold in different ways depending on the types of obsessions and rituals involved. They also play out differently within different types of relationships. For example, if the person you love with OCD is a child, you will feel and react differently than if she is an adolescent or an adult. If the person is your son, things will go differently than if it's your spouse or partner. In this chapter, I'll help you understand how these interpersonal patterns work, which will provide a foundation for using the strategies I describe later in this book to thoughtfully remove yourself from the OCD cycle so that you're able to normalize your life and provide a healthier kind of support for your loved one.

Accommodation: When Others "Help" with OCD

When something happens to a loved one—your spouse, partner, sibling, child, or parent—everyone else in the household has to adjust so that the family or relationship can function as well as possible. Think about it: if your son broke his leg, you and other family members would step in to relieve him of some of his chores and responsibilities while he was immobilized. Hopefully, your family would also provide emotional support to let him know he is loved and cared for. Generally, this kind of adjustment makes good sense and is a healthy way for family members to react. But if you're not careful, it could also have some unintended negative effects. Let's say that to regain strength in his leg, your son now requires a lot of physical exercise. If family members have taken over his chores while he was inactive and they continue to do them for him, he might not have the opportunity to get the exercise he now needs.

The same thing can happen when a loved one has OCD. In one way or another, the family makes adjustments to help manage the obsessional fears, avoidance patterns, and rituals. A husband pays the bills so his wife doesn't have to worry about making mistakes. A mother leaves work early so she can drive her adult daughter to the hairdresser because of her obsessional fears that she'll hit a pedestrian. The rest of the family is ready to leave the house but waits around for one child when she gets stuck turning off light switches and checking that all appliances are unplugged. When a loved one gets anxious and you know what will lower the anxiety, the first instinct is to step in and do whatever is needed to keep this anxiety in check. It might be an important way to show your loved one how much you care about her. At other times, the person with OCD is so uncomfortable that she lets others know (sometimes in a demanding way) what she needs them to do to help minimize her anxiety.

Of course, protecting someone from situations that are *actually dangerous* is healthy and appropriate. But as you know, obsessional fears are based on exaggerated estimates of threat. Changing your routine to protect a loved one unnecessarily from obsessional fear, as if an actual threat existed, is what we call *accommodation*. It is not only unnecessary but can have negative consequences.

What Does Accommodation Look Like?

Let's look at the patterns of accommodation in the four people with OCD introduced in Chapter 1. In Eduardo's family, accommodation became a full-time job for his mother, yet his sister and father also made adjustments:

> When Eduardo was 12, his mother started cleaning the toilet for him every morning because of his fear of "toilet germs." And later, when he became afraid that other people could spread toilet germs anywhere in the house, his mother took to cleaning wherever Eduardo wanted to go. Eduardo's father and sister also had special instructions not to touch certain things, such as the remote control or refrigerator door, unless they first used hand sanitizer. It had become part of the family routine to keep everything super clean for Eduardo, including certain parts of the family car. When Eduardo noticed that his father and sister were sometimes breaking these "rules," he began retreating to his room for safety. This happened more and more until one day he refused to come out. At that point, his mother agreed to prepare all of his meals and bring them to his room—which Eduardo would accept only if she had used hand sanitizer first. His father also set up a computer and gaming system for Eduardo's room so he would be comfortable staying there all the time. His mom even quit her job so she could stay home and provide homeschooling. Eduardo only let his mother into his room if she had showered first. His mother also did Eduardo's laundry, cleaned his room, and made his bed every day.

Ariel's situation was a little different since she was an adult with a spouse (Ben) and two kids:

> Ariel's worrying about break-ins, fires, and floods began shortly after she married Ben and moved into their new home. But when her daughters were born, her obsessions went into overdrive. There was a nightly ritual of sitting down to have Ben explain that he'd locked every door and turned off every faucet and electrical appliance. After a while, this wasn't enough, and she made Ben walk around the house with her to check everything. Ben knew he had to accompany Ariel on these

checks and even keep a written log of all the checking; otherwise Ariel would worry that he'd forgotten something and the ritual would have to be repeated. Occasionally, while at work, Ariel would call Ben at his job and beg him to run home to check that she'd locked all the doors or turned off all the appliances before she'd left the house. He complied because he knew it was the only way to calm Ariel down. After several of these episodes, the couple planned their daily schedules so that Ben would usually be the last to leave the house for work. This way, Ariel didn't have to feel anxious about being responsible for locking up and making sure everything was off.

Xavier was an adult living at home with his parents. Here's how his father and mother accommodated his OCD symptoms related to religion:

After 2 years of college, Xavier dropped out, worked in a furniture store, and lived on his own. That's when he started obsessing about God and calling his parents to ask questions such as "Do you think I'm faithful enough?" and "How do I know if I fully appreciate God?" Xavier's father spent a great deal of time on the phone every evening trying to reassure Xavier that everything was fine between him and God. Occasionally, the anxiety would be so intense that Xavier would spend entire days reading the Bible or searching online for answers to his questions. Eventually, he missed so much work (and had so much trouble concentrating when he was present) that he was fired. Xavier's parents reached out to help him find treatment for OCD, but Xavier insisted he didn't have any problems. His parents thought it was best if Xavier moved back home with them—that was 10 years ago, and Xavier has been living at home and completely dependent on his parents ever since. His parents provide everything Xavier wants and are happy to take time to discuss religion, sin, faith, and God. Nightly discussions in which they reassure Xavier that he hasn't done anything sinful last for several hours at a time. Xavier is technically employed at his father's hardware store but shows up for work only when he feels "up to it." Although this arrangement seems to work for everyone in the house, Xavier's parents would much prefer that Xavier get help so he can move out and be independent. But when they bring up this issue, Xavier gets angry and says that things are fine.

Linda's husband, Nicholas, played a large role in accommodating Linda's OCD symptoms:

Linda and Nicholas had a healthy marriage for over 30 years. They were excited to become grandparents for the first time when Emma was born. When Linda began having intrusive sexual thoughts, they didn't want to tell their son and daughter-in-law because of the embarrassment, so Nicholas started making up excuses for why Linda couldn't visit the baby and why Emma couldn't come to their home either. Nicholas also hated seeing his wife struggle with such terrible thoughts, so he went along with Linda's idea to avoid any reminders of Emma. Somewhat reluctantly, he agreed not to mention her to Linda and to remove all pictures of Emma from their home. Every time sexual thoughts about Emma did come up, he reassured Linda that she wasn't a pedophile and that he'd actually had similar thoughts but didn't give them any weight. When Linda insisted that the couple refrain from watching any TV shows or movies that were in any way sexually suggestive and stick to watching only things that Linda deemed "wholesome," Nicholas started to feel that things were going too far— although he never let Linda see his frustration. He went along with her wishes to protect her from the obsessions, even though it meant missing out on his favorite shows.

Later in this chapter we'll delve more deeply into what drives accommodation and the negative consequences it has. For now, consider the three ways you might be accommodating your relative's OCD.

Getting Involved in Rituals

At some point, most relatives who live in the same household with a person who has OCD find themselves participating in rituals to help their loved one control or avoid anxiety. A father might help his daughter with fears of making mistakes check all of her e-mails several times before she sends them. A wife might shower before having sex with her husband because she knows it reduces his fear of contamination. As you read, Ben was involved in Ariel's checking and reassurance-seeking rituals: sometimes he checked for her, and at other times he reassured her that she'd already checked.

It is also accommodation if you're facilitating rituals, such as:

- Driving a relative back home to use the bathroom in the middle of an outing to the mall
- Taking your child to the hardware store so she can seek reassurance

from an "expert" salesperson about the dangers of using a certain chemical

- Supplying your loved one with extra time or items needed to perform rituals.

A mother I once worked with would postpone her errands for hours while her son completed extensive tapping rituals before leaving the house. Some parents stock up on large quantities of soap, detergents, or toilet paper so their child can perform excessive washing, cleaning, or toileting routines. Similarly, giving an adult gas money to help offset the cost of rituals that involve extra driving fits into this category. A related form of accommodation is to provide excuses to other people for a loved one's rituals, like when Eduardo's mother would call school to say that Eduardo had the flu even though it was his lengthy showering and toilet rituals that kept him stuck in the bathroom for hours. It would be impossible for me to list *all* possible forms of accommodation—indeed the possibilities are endless. What's important to know is that accommodation occurs when you make it easier for the person with OCD to perform rituals.

Getting Involved in Avoidance

Another common form of accommodation involves allowing (or putting up with), assisting, or supporting your family member's avoidance behavior. This might involve directly helping with avoidance, such as when Ben agreed to leave the house after Ariel so that she wouldn't feel accountable for locking up. It might also involve making it easier for a loved one to continue avoidance, such as when Nicholas would "cover" for Linda by telling their family that she was sick when in fact she was avoiding Emma because of obsessions. Couples may also avoid doing certain things together so that the partner with OCD doesn't have to face feared situations or thoughts. A good example of this is Linda and Nicholas's mutual avoidance of certain TV shows.

Here are some other examples:

- A family agrees not to go to a particular movie theater because one family member is afraid the seats are contaminated.
- A husband agrees to keep knives and other items that could be used as weapons (such as a hammer or baseball bat) out of sight so that they don't trigger his spouse's obsessional thoughts of violence.
- A mother makes her adult son's bed and washes his sheets and

underwear every morning so he doesn't have to worry about contact with bedsheets or clothing he fears might be contaminated from wet dreams.

- A brother agrees not to have certain friends visit the house because his sister with OCD fears they will bring germs into the home.

- A family routinely ends their outings early (or cancels them altogether) so the daughter can avoid having to use public bathrooms.

In one of the more extreme examples that I've encountered, a husband switched jobs because his wife, who had obsessional fears of the herpes virus, once saw a woman with a cold sore enter the store where he had been working. The wife was constantly worried that her husband would "bring herpes home" if he continued to work there.

Changing Up Family Routines

Another form of accommodation occurs when family routines, schedules, plans, and other activity patterns or household responsibilities become dictated by OCD. Take Eduardo's family as an example. His mother quit her job so she could stay at home to take care of Eduardo. But this meant his father now had to work longer hours. Eduardo's parents decided this new arrangement was worthwhile because they felt they needed to minimize Eduardo's anxiety. Similarly, Xavier's parents accommodated by allowing Xavier to live in their home. They provided him with whatever he needed and stayed up late at night to give him reassurance. It was also accommodation to keep Xavier on the payroll at the hardware store and allow him to frequently miss work simply because he didn't "feel up to it." This truly inconvenienced his father, something most employers wouldn't put up with. Xavier was also permitted to shirk his responsibilities around the house, such as daily chores, if he was feeling too anxious. If the typical routines in your family—living or sleeping arrangements, social plans, child care responsibilities, homework, chores, family outings, trips, or just relaxing—are modified or put on hold because of OCD, it's considered accommodation.

Because of Linda's obsessional fears, she and her husband decided that their favorite television shows were off limits. They restricted their viewing to "wholesome" channels such as the Food Network or the History Channel. Another couple agreed that the husband (with OCD) would sleep in a separate room from his wife because of upsetting obsessional thoughts about impulsively harming her while she slept. Each evening, she complied with his request to be locked in his room so he wouldn't "escape and do anything ter-rible" during the night. A family I worked with ate only at restaurants that had been given a perfect score on their health inspection due to one family mem-ber's fears of food poisoning. Finally, despite being perfectly happy with their church, Xavier's parents agreed to switch their place of worship because of Xavier's obsessional fear that it wasn't conservative enough for God's liking.

Accommodation in Your Own Family or Relationship

Accommodation is so common that it's not so much a matter of *if* but rather *how* and *how much* it happens in your family or relationship. In what ways do you help your loved one avoid becoming anxious? What do (or don't) you do as a family just to avoid the anxiety? How have family members taken over tasks and responsibilities for the person with OCD? How do you and others participate in rituals? For many families, the problem is that accommodation becomes routine, so family members don't even think about it anymore. In other words, you might not even realize how you've fallen into these patterns. And if your goal is to end accommodation, you'll have a hard time if you don't know when and how it's happening. That's why in Chapter 8 of this book I'll help you take stock of the accommodation in your family or relationship.

For now, think about how you (and others) respond to your loved one's OCD symptoms. What do you do for him (or allow to happen) that you wouldn't do (or allow) if he didn't have OCD? Would you do these things for someone else in your family who doesn't have OCD? If the answer is no, then it's likely that accommodation is occurring. You can also ask yourself if you would prefer to stop the behavior in question. Most of the time, accom-modation feels at least somewhat excessive or unnecessary. So, even though your intent is to protect your loved one, if there's a part of you that feels like you're pushing the limits of what's appropriate, it's likely that you've identified accommodation behavior.

Accommodation: Protective but Ineffective

Isn't it the right thing to do to clean Eduardo's room for him if he's so anxious about germs? Shouldn't Ben help Ariel check at night if it calms and reassures her? Aren't Xavier's parents just being good caregivers by providing for their son and protecting him from anxiety? Isn't it just the compassionate thing to do for Nicholas to protect Linda from unwanted sexual thoughts? Anxiety, after all, can seem unbearable. Uncertainty can seem agonizing. And isn't it dreadful to have upsetting intrusive thoughts running through your head?

We don't like seeing our loved ones in an anxious or distressed state, much less facing danger. So it's only natural to want to protect them if there's anything we can do to keep them safe or at ease. Accommodation, therefore, comes from a good place. Helping your family member with OCD avoid or reduce anxiety might be a way of saying "I love you" or "I'm concerned about you." These actions might have become patterns that you or your family just do because you care. At other times, the person with OCD might let you know when she needs help reducing obsessions and anxiety. Sometimes this takes on a demanding or threatening tone, and you know that if you don't help, your loved one will become angry. But whether it is out of concern or to avoid a negative interaction, accommodation helps alleviate distress in the moment. And it's easy to see some good in this.

But as the heading of this section suggests, despite being mostly well intentioned on your part, accommodation actually ends up working against you *and* your loved one with OCD in the long run. Let's explore how this happens in more detail.

Accommodation fuels the vicious cycle of OCD. Research shows that there's a link between accommodation and more severe OCD symptoms. This is true for kids, teens, and grown-ups living with their families, as well as within adult couples in which one partner has OCD. Accommodation plays into the vicious cycle I described in Chapter 2 in a few ways. For one thing, it doesn't matter whether the rituals or avoidance behaviors are being performed by your loved one alone or with help from others. When an obsessional trigger is avoided or a ritual is performed, it reduces anxiety in the short term but makes OCD stronger in the long run. That's because accommodation robs your relative of the opportunity to learn that (1) the disastrous outcomes she fears are unlikely and (2) she *can* manage the anxious feelings and unwanted obsessional thoughts.

To make matters worse, the more others accommodate, the more your family member feels that he's not capable of functioning without the accommodation. This is a vicious cycle of its own: if you consistently act on your loved one's behalf, handling difficult situations for him, he never gets the opportunity to learn how to handle such situations for himself. This reduces his self-confidence, and he'll feel like he can't do without the help. This is also how many families get stuck in accommodation patterns that snowball over months and years. Not only that, accommodation sends the (false) message that anxiety and obsessional thoughts are harmful and dangerous and that avoidance and rituals are necessary to prevent catastrophe. Think about it: if those around you are always working to protect you from something you fear, it would only reinforce your belief that danger is present.

Accommodation reduces the incentive to change. Eduardo's parents were perplexed when Eduardo refused to get help for his OCD. Wasn't he sick of being afraid of germs (pun intended), being stuck in his room, and having to do so many compulsive rituals? Xavier's parents were also surprised that Xavier was so opposed to getting help. Didn't he want to overcome his scrupulosity, become more independent, and have a family of his own? I've counseled many couples and families in which the person with OCD is being pushed to seek treatment by the same caregivers who are accommodating their symptoms. The outcome is usually predictable: the person with OCD pushes back—often strongly—and rejects getting needed help. Let's look at why this happens:

When family members *without* OCD change their routines to accommodate OCD symptoms, it makes it easier for the person *with* OCD to live with the disorder. Think about it: although Eduardo had OCD, his life was actually quite comfortable. He didn't have to attend school, make his bed, clean his room, fix food for himself, or have other responsibilities and obligations that many 17-year-olds commonly have. He stayed in his room all day while his mother waited on him hand and foot. His parents even got him a computer and video games for his room! So in relieving Eduardo of the weight of OCD, his parents had taken on this burden themselves. Is it any wonder Eduardo had little desire to get help? Of course, the situation wasn't ideal, but it was good enough as far as he was concerned (although certainly not if you asked his parents!). Can you see how the same pattern developed in Xavier's family? Xavier didn't have to worry about working or other responsibilities since his parents took care of everything. OCD was really *their* problem. How much did Xavier have to gain by getting treatment?

Maybe you appreciate how much Eduardo's and Xavier's parents did to protect their sons from discomfort. But for all their hard work, they were frustrated by their sons' lack of motivation to get help. They didn't understand the dynamic here: the same accommodation that protected their sons from becoming anxious also kept them from wanting to put forth the effort to get help. That's one reason I want to help you reduce your accommodation. When you (and other family members) are no longer protecting your loved one from the pain of OCD, he has something to gain by getting help. In later chapters I'll give you the tools you need to change the ways you interact with your loved one around OCD. Don't worry, the aim is not to disrupt your sense of closeness. I certainly want you to be emotionally supportive when your family member is feeling anxious; but I'll help you do so without accommodating.

Accommodation harms relationships. Sure, Ben didn't like seeing Ariel so worried about break-ins and fires, but do you think he was happy about all that he had to do to keep Ariel from worrying? Checking the doors and appliances every night—*after* giving Ariel loads of verbal reassurance—was extremely irritating to him. More and more, he found himself losing his patience and his temper with Ariel. He would snap at her, "What's wrong with you!? We go through this same routine every night! When will you get a clue that I care about safety too? I'm not going to leave the doors unlocked! Why don't you trust me?"

Similarly, even though Nicholas wanted to keep Linda from having sexual thoughts about Emma, he was annoyed about all the sacrifices he was making just to protect her from these senseless obsessions. He felt left out when his friends and their families would all get together and spend time sharing stories and pictures of their grandchildren. And although he never told Linda, Nicholas strongly resented her for making him miss out on what was supposed to be a joyful stage of life. He didn't feel emotionally close to her; and intimacy was out of the question.

Think back on all the time and energy you've spent trying to protect your loved one from anxiety. Maybe it's relatively minor adjustments that you've made, or maybe you and others have gone to great lengths to accommodate the OCD. But how much satisfaction do you really get from knowing how much you've put yourself out for your loved one? How much does your loved one appreciate your efforts? The truth is that accommodation is usually a "one-way street." You're doing all the hard work for your loved one and getting little or nothing in return. And unfortunately, that's a recipe for stressful and dissatisfying relationships.

How Does Your Loved One Get You to Accommodate?

Perhaps you've recognized the futility of accommodation and refused to comply with your loved one's avoidance and rituals or his insistence that you follow the OCD-based rules he's imposed. But this can also lead to conflict.

There were mornings when Eduardo and his mother would be screaming at each other in the bathroom because she wasn't cleaning the toilet and shower to Eduardo's satisfaction. She would try to explain, saying "I've

done the best I can, but we've been in here for almost an hour already.
I'm going downstairs to make breakfast for your father and sister."
Eduardo would become furious. "No! How can you just leave me here
like this, you bitch!?" His mother would yell back at him, "Don't talk
to me that way! You're not the only one who lives in this house, you
know!" That's when Eduardo would play the suicide card: "You don't
care about me! I swear, if you leave I'll take all my pills and kill myself!"
Then Eduardo's mother would throw in the towel. She simply couldn't
stand the thought of her son in so much distress that he was thinking
of suicide. What if he actually went through with it!? She would end up
succumbing to Eduardo's demands every time he mentioned harming
himself.

Although not always to such extremes, this is a common pattern that unfolds in families and intimate relationships affected by OCD. It's also another reason that accommodation is so difficult to stop. Isn't it easier to just give in and accommodate than to put up with tantrums, intimidation, or emotional blackmail? That's what your loved one is banking on when she turns to threats and drama. Later in this book I'll give you helpful strategies for effectively responding to and getting out of this cycle.

It's easy to look at this kind of behavior and see it as controlling. And, yes, your loved one does it to get you to accommodate to her OCD. But before going any further, it's important to also see it from your family member's point of view. For the most part, her escalation in emotion, threats, or intimidation occurs because she's afraid something awful will happen if you don't help with rituals or other forms of accommodation. In other words, she's not just trying to get your attention, control you, or make you upset just for kicks. To her, the situation seems overwhelming or dangerous, and she's just doing what she thinks will get you to help her feel safe.

Research suggests that it's *mothers,* as opposed to fathers, siblings, or spouses, who are most likely to be targeted with this sort of coercion. Yet any family member can become a recipient, and I've come across a multitude of ways that people with OCD—both young and old—attempt to pressure others into helping with (or putting up with) rituals, avoidance, or other strategies for minimizing anxiety. Younger children are most likely to resort to tantrums, whereas older children and adults tend to use more creative approaches. These might include intimidation with threats of force or violence, the actual use of force or violence, verbal abuse or accusations (such as "you don't care about me"), and threats of recklessness, self-harm, or suicide.

Adults and older children might also engage in patterns of highly upsetting or disruptive behavior that pushes (or exceeds) established limits with the goal of coercing others into accommodating. Your adult son with obsessional fears of dirty laundry stops showering and changing his clothes (so that his body odor becomes unbearable) until you agree to wash his laundry separately from that of the rest of the family. Your teenaged daughter who is afraid of food poisoning refuses to eat because she disapproves of the way you clean the dishes and silverware. Your adult child continually deprives you of sleep by knocking on the bedroom door until you answer his reassurance-seeking questions. Your partner or spouse withholds sex or other forms of intimacy because of your reluctance to accommodate to her compulsive need for certain things to be organized just right. In later chapters you'll learn healthy and supportive ways to respond to these fear-driven behaviors so you don't feel as if your back is against the wall.

What's Happening to Your Happy Home?

I probably don't have to tell you that living with OCD, and the stress of accommodating its demands, can transform your home from sanctuary to battle zone. Many families get caught in endless arguments over how OCD is affecting their routines and relationships. And OCD can take up so much time or curtail family activities to such a great extent that opportunities for enjoyable interactions are few and far between. Even if you're all too familiar with the negative impact OCD is having on your family, it's important to take a closer look at the ways OCD interferes, because it will provide you with avenues for change that can ease OCD's grip on your family. Here are the patterns that can result when OCD affects families and relationships.

Passivity. This means being ineffective at standing up for yourself. Eduardo's mother, for example, was passive when it came to saying no to helping Eduardo with avoidance and rituals. She knew that her accommodation went far beyond what parents typically do for their teenage sons but didn't know how to tell Eduardo no. When you become passive, you're likely to feel taken advantage of, as Eduardo's mother often felt. Eduardo could ask for almost anything, and she would usually agree. And if she didn't, he could raise his voice, call her nasty names, and make threats—and then she'd respond. What's more, Eduardo was never punished for his unacceptable behavior, so there was no incentive to stop his tantrums. Eduardo's mother was at her wit's end but didn't have the skills to make the necessary changes. Does passivity lead to stress in your family or relationship?

Avoidance. In this context, avoidance is a communication pattern in which you shy away from sharing your opinions, discussing difficult topics, and solving problems in your relationships. Maybe you avoid conflict or tend to be indecisive. Perhaps you constantly struggle with wanting to please others. The problem with avoidant communication is that it often leaves you feeling like you've not gotten what you wanted, which can make you blame yourself. Then, when things finally come to a head, you boil over with anger at your loved one with OCD. Take Linda's husband, Nicholas. He avoided telling Linda how frustrated he was that OCD was dictating their lives until something would happen and he couldn't hold it in any longer. Then he'd explode in a fit of range.

Interdependency. This refers to a relationship in which one person "needs" the other, who in turn needs to be needed. Take Xavier's relationship with his parents. On one hand, Xavier "needed" to be living with his parents because they took care of many responsibilities for him and gave him reassurance. Yet at the same time, his parents—especially his mother—also "needed" Xavier. Even though she wished he was free of OCD and off on his own, Mom also got some fulfilment from her role as his caregiver. A part of her was content to spend hours each day providing reassurance for Xavier because it made her feel needed. The problem is that interdependency—which can occur between adults as well as between adults and their children—is difficult to get out of and often leads to depression, self-blame, denial of problems, and resisting help. In Chapter 7 you'll learn ways to practice healthier, supportive communication patterns for dealing with OCD.

Arguments. It seems simple enough: if your loved one has an irrational fear, just use logic and reason to help her get over it. No doubt you've been down this road . . . and seen that it doesn't work. Still, the senselessness of your loved one's obsessional fears and rituals makes it extremely difficult to resist giving lectures, engaging in debates, having arguments about the seeming illogic of her anxiety, or demanding (perhaps in a hostile manner) that she see things your way and "snap out of it." But it's not for a lack of trying that you can't get your relative to change her mind. The truth is you won't win these arguments no matter what you do. Your loved one has reasons for being afraid, and those reasons might not conform to the same logic you're using. Sure, it's extremely frustrating to you; but what's worse is that when you debate, you're only helping her come up with more reasons to dig her heels in and defend her irrational fears and rituals. So at best, arguing with your loved one and insisting on change elevates the general level of stress in your family or relationship. At worst, it also strengthens her OCD.

Recall that one of Xavier's obsessions, when he was younger, was that his girlfriend, Alyssa, might have become pregnant and then had an abortion without Xavier knowing. Xavier never had sex with Alyssa but did get an erection while fully dressed and kissing her. Even years later, Xavier would ask his parents to reassure him that there was no pregnancy and no abortion. As you might imagine, his parents couldn't resist trying to use logic to put the matter to rest once and for all. Sometimes they were critical of Xavier as well:

XAVIER'S FATHER: Xavier, you're being ridiculous. If you were both fully clothed, you couldn't have had sex with Alyssa. What's wrong with you that you can't understand that?

XAVIER: But I think I got an erection. What if my fly was unzipped and my penis stuck out?

XAVIER'S FATHER: What about Alyssa? Her pants and underwear?

XAVIER: I just feel like I can't remember for sure. What if we took off our clothes and I forgot? I have to know.

XAVIER'S FATHER: I'm telling you. You're not making any sense. There's no logical way it could have happened. And you would remember if you two had sex. I really can't believe you're afraid of this. It's completely silly.

Of course, this strategy failed to convince Xavier. In fact, it made him think of new things to obsess about and worry about—maybe he *did* get undressed with Alyssa but forgot about this "detail" as well. When you engage in logical arguments with a loved one, you play into OCD symptoms and increase the overall level of interpersonal stress.

So, what can you do instead? How can you change the rules laid down by OCD to free your family from its trap? Is there a way to help free your loved one who is suffering from the disorder as well?

Fortunately, there is a lot of research evidence—and a lot of experience compiled by many mental health professionals—that certain treatments are very effective for OCD. Unfortunately, and as you may already know, those with OCD may resist the changes required by these strategies. They may refuse to seek professional help or reject the idea of using self-help methods to extricate themselves from the OCD trap. But *you* can still use the principles and strategies in these treatments to release yourself from the patterns of accommodation and the family conflicts that are getting you down. As I've found in my years of practice and research, applying these methods—which you'll learn about in the next chapter—within your family sometimes has the happy benefit of helping the person with OCD as well.

4

Treatment That Can Help Your Relative—and Your Family

I have devoted the first three chapters of this book to helping you understand how OCD operates because it sets the stage for understanding how we help people overcome OCD. Knowing how obsessions and compulsions trap your relative—and end up ensnaring you too—will make it easier to see how treatment can break the vicious cycle. It turns out that the treatment scientifically proven to be most effective for OCD overall is also best able to disentangle you from OCD and help you provide the best possible support to your loved one. And that treatment is cognitive-behavioral therapy (CBT). Understanding the techniques of CBT, the rationale behind them, and the role of family in this therapy is an important initial step in reducing accommodation, communicating better with your loved one, and improving how you feel about this person, your family, and yourself. And even if your relative is not currently in treatment, when *you* use CBT methods to stop playing by OCD's rules, your relative just might decide that it's time to try therapy.

What Is CBT?

CBT is a skills-based approach to treatment in which the therapist and patient work together to develop an understanding of the problem and create a treatment plan that involves learning and practicing healthier ways of thinking, behaving, and coping with life. You can think of a CBT therapist as a sort of coach or teacher. She helps patients become their own therapists by teaching them skills in the session and then assigning "homework" practice to reinforce what was learned.

CBT includes a wide range of techniques and methods based on the core principle that psychological problems and disorders stem, in large part, from (1) faulty or unhelpful ways of thinking (*cognitions*) and (2) learned patterns of problematic *behavior*. In OCD, CBT trains the patient to recognize the problematic ways of thinking discussed in Chapter 2, replace them with healthier thinking patterns, and change behavior (such as performing rituals) that keeps OCD in charge. Across decades of research, studies show that CBT is associated with a 60–70% reduction in OCD symptoms for about 60–70% of people, with sustained improvements over the long term.

How Is CBT Used for OCD?

The main "ingredients" in effective CBT for OCD are *exposure* and *response prevention*. *Exposure therapy* is the process of deliberately confronting fear triggers to learn that they're generally safe and therefore don't need to be avoided. *Response prevention* means refraining from rituals to learn that these behaviors aren't necessary to prevent feared outcomes. In the 1960s, psychologist Victor Meyer developed a learning-based therapy in which he helped patients with OCD (1) confront the very situations and thoughts that provoked their obsessional fear and (2) refrain from doing their compulsive rituals. For example, Meyer helped people with contamination obsessions deliberately touch objects that triggered their fears of becoming ill and then abstain from all washing and cleaning so they could go on feeling "contaminated."

Of course, Dr. Meyer realized this process would initially make his patients *more* anxious, but he wanted them to learn for themselves what would happen when they remained exposed to obsessional fear triggers for a long time without ritualizing away their anxiety. As he had hoped, his patients' anxiety and obsessional thoughts didn't spiral out of control or lead to any harmful effects. In fact, the patients felt emboldened because they learned (1) that they could tolerate anxious thoughts and feelings until they eventually subsided on their own and (2) that their fears were exaggerated. Those with contamination obsessions, for example, learned they were very unlikely to become ill, which helped disprove their fears of germs and sickness. As a result, they began to see their once-feared situations as safe. When patients repeated this process daily over a few months, their urges to perform compulsive rituals dissipated, which allowed them more time and freedom to get their lives back on track.

For over 50 years now, researchers and clinicians around the world (including me and my team) have been working to refine and improve this therapy and adapt it for all different manifestations of obsessions and rituals. Today, exposure and response prevention (or "ERP" for short) is available in both standard outpatient (usually 16–20 weekly therapy sessions) and intensive outpatient (15 weekday sessions over 3 weeks) formats, as well as in partial hospitalization and residential programs. There are also numerous self-help books, Internet-based programs, and smartphone applications available based on ERP (you'll learn about the pros and cons of these approaches in Chapter 14). And two additional CBT techniques, cognitive therapy and acceptance and commitment therapy (ACT), are sometimes used along with ERP.

State-of-the-Art CBT for OCD

CBT for OCD includes the techniques summarized in the box below. I'll go into more detail about the sequence that treatment typically follows in Chapter 15 in case your relative is considering entering treatment and you both want to know what to expect. Here I'm going to summarize how the

---

Summary of Effective CBT Techniques for Treating OCD

Technique	Aims and goals
Situational exposure	Practice engaging with situations and items that trigger obsessional fear to learn that they, and the fear itself, are safe and manageable
Imaginal exposure	Practice engaging with obsessional thoughts, images, anxiety, and uncertainty to learn that these mental experiences are safe and tolerable
Response prevention	Practice resisting rituals to learn that they are not necessary for remaining safe and managing fear
Cognitive therapy	Correct faulty thinking patterns that lead to the misinterpretation of obsessional thoughts and overestimates of threat
Acceptance and commitment therapy	Learn healthier ways of interacting with obsessions and anxiety to improve quality of life

techniques work, which will help you apply them to supporting your relative and ending accommodation.

Exposure

There are two types of exposure, situational and imaginal, to address obsessional fears about external situations as well as mental obsessions.

Situational exposure. In either professional or self-help CBT, one of the first steps is to make a list of all the situations, objects, thoughts, and images that provoke obsessional fear in your relative. Situational exposure is a technique that will help your relative engage with the external stimuli that she's been avoiding. Usually, a new exposure task from her situational exposure list is introduced at each session (as agreed upon by your relative and therapist) and the therapist coaches your relative through it. Your family member will also practice each exposure independently (for "homework") between sessions.

For situational exposure to work, the person needs to remain in the feared situation long enough to (1) correct mistaken beliefs about the dangerousness of the situation and (2) prove that feelings of anxiety and fear are safe and manageable. Learning that anxiety itself isn't something to be afraid of is an important part of doing exposure because it helps your loved one build confidence. Not only that, anxiety and fear are likely to *decrease* naturally when situational exposure lasts long enough and is repeated over and over—a result called *habituation*.

Most types of obsessions lend themselves well to situational exposure. Exposures for contamination fears, for example, involve touching "contaminated" objects such as garbage cans, money, or door knobs and going to feared situations or places such as public restrooms. For obsessions about accidents that are triggered by driving near pedestrians, exposure to driving past people on roadways would be helpful. Similarly, for obsessions about violence or religion, exposure might entail watching horror movies or confronting unlucky numbers, knives, Bibles, or religious symbols that provoke anxiety.

Think about the kinds of situational exposures that might help Eduardo get past his fear of "bathroom germs." If he touched items in the bathroom and spread the "contamination" to his own room and his things, he would learn that such germs are unlikely to make him ill. Similarly, if Ariel used her stove or iron—which she'd been avoiding—she would learn that these appliances are unlikely to burn down her house. For his exposures, Xavier might try praying while distracted, or even skipping or mispronouncing a word or two. He could also tell that funny, though a bit off-color, joke that he recently heard. And helpful exposures for Linda would involve watching the shows she'd been avoiding, looking at pictures of Emma, going to Emma's home, and interacting with her. In fact, Linda should probably practice changing the baby's diaper and giving her a bath for exposure.

Imaginal exposure. What if your relative's obsession is about murdering someone, going to hell, or spreading illness to other people? Obviously, it's neither practical nor ethical to do situational exposure to these kinds of things. This is where *imaginal exposure* comes in. Imaginal exposure involves engaging with mental pictures of obsessional thoughts that provoke fear. Similar to situational exposure, the goal is to learn that thinking about these obsessional thoughts is not dangerous (however unpleasant they may feel). Also similar to situational exposure, imaginal exposure initially provokes anxiety, and with repeated practice it usually results in habituation. But one has to actually go toe to toe with an obsession to find out that the distress is temporary and manageable. The analogy I think of is that of a horror movie: watch it for the first time and you feel tense and frightened; but watch it 50 times and it loses it punch.

So, although Ariel wouldn't actually start a fire for therapy, she might write a story in which she's mistakenly left the stove on and comes back from work to find her home ablaze. Her therapist would then want her to leave home and practice reading the story *without going back to check* (as we'll see in the next section). Similarly, Xavier could imagine that God was upset with him for telling a dirty joke. Finally, while changing Emma's diaper, Linda could deliberately think about touching her granddaughter's private parts. The goal is for your relative to develop more self-confidence by learning that although these thoughts, images, and ideas are distressing, they're not signs of actual danger—they're just mental noise.

Response Prevention

In addition to provoking anxiety, situational and imaginal exposure trigger the urge to perform rituals. But exposure that's followed by rituals just perpetuates the vicious cycle. If Eduardo sat in a family chair and handled the TV remote control for situational exposure but then afterward took a shower and changed his clothes, he wouldn't learn that the chair and the remote are safe, or that he can manage the feelings of anxiety that exposure provokes. He might even (mis)attribute not getting sick to his rituals and continue to be afraid of these items. This is exactly why exposure must be accompanied by *response prevention,* which means resisting urges to do rituals. For Eduardo, this would mean refraining from washing, cleaning, changing clothes, and the like. For Ariel, this means stopping her checking and reassurance-seeking rituals. For Xavier, response prevention would entail refraining from asking his parents for reassurance.

Keep in mind that the term *response prevention* isn't exactly accurate— we don't ever physically *prevent* anyone from doing rituals in CBT. Rather, the therapist coaches the person with OCD to make the decision to resist urges to do rituals. And while cessation of *all* rituals is the eventual goal, this doesn't mean your relative needs to go "cold turkey" and stop them all at once. Rituals can be gradually reduced or modified in ways that make them less potent before they are ultimately dropped. The therapist and your loved one will collaboratively decide on a strategy or "road map" for response prevention, and your relative will keep track of how well she can stick to the plan so that extra attention can be dedicated to trouble spots.

Cognitive Therapy

As you've already seen, thoughts and beliefs play an important role in OCD. Eduardo *misjudged* the probability and seriousness of contamination from "bathroom germs." Ariel *overestimated* the risk of fires and felt an inflated sense of responsibility for making sure they never occurred. Xavier *believed* he couldn't tolerate uncertainty about his previous behavior and relationship with God. Linda *misinterpreted* her senseless sexual thoughts as meaning that there was something terribly wrong with her. The importance of these faulty cognitions is why ERP may be augmented with *cognitive therapy*—a set of tools for recognizing and correcting the kinds of errors in thinking that overlie obsessions and rituals.

Cognitive therapy usually involves the person with OCD and the therapist working together to carefully examine faulty cognitive patterns and come up with more useful, logical, and *correct* cognitions. Sometimes this involves "experiments" (which might be similar to exposure practices) to test out whether fears come true. Cognitive therapy can help people think more carefully when they become anxious, and it can therefore provide a strong foundation for doing ERP. But I do not recommend cognitive therapy on its own as a treatment for OCD.

Acceptance and Commitment Therapy (ACT)

ACT (pronounced "act") is an intervention that helps your relative become more *open* and *willing* to experience obsessions and anxiety (without having to resist, control, or fight them) so these private experiences don't interfere with important parts of his life. A therapist might, for example, help Linda develop a healthier and more accepting relationship with her OCD-related thoughts so that she's not locked in a constant battle with them. Ariel might focus on simply observing her obsessions, rather than responding to them as if they're facts. Xavier might be encouraged to identify the things he values in life that have been affected by OCD and practice pursuing what he values instead of allowing obsessions and anxiety to derail these activities. ACT relies heavily on the use of metaphors to guide therapeutic discussion; and because it is consistent with the goals of ERP, it's often used along with these techniques.

When Is CBT Less Effective?

Although CBT is helpful for most people with OCD, there are certain factors that can interfere with treatment response. It's important to be aware of these factors at this point because they can also make it trickier to become disentangled from your loved one's OCD. If any of the following factors affect your relative, I recommend that you move forward with the program in this book after consulting with a mental health professional.

Severe depression. Depression is often accompanied by hopelessness, helplessness, and a lack of interest in enjoyable activities. With depression, there's also a higher risk of self-harm. I'm not saying it won't be successful, but all of these symptoms *can* interfere with the effects of CBT as well as your efforts to use the strategies you'll read about later in this book. Therefore, I recommend discussing your plans with a professional.

Psychosis or bipolar disorder. If your loved one with OCD also has a psychotic disorder (for instance, schizophrenia) or bipolar disorder, and her symptoms are not currently well-managed (for example, with the help of appropriate medications), they might restrict her ability to learn from the changes I'll be suggesting you make. It will therefore be important to address these other problems before you work toward becoming disentangled from OCD.

Attentional or executive functioning problems. Attention deficit disorder and problems with memory, flexible thinking, or self-control can hinder the ability to function independently—especially for children. If your relative with OCD also has one of these problems, it might require that you modify some of the advice I provide in later chapters. Working with a qualified professional (see Chapter 14 if your loved one doesn't already have a provider) will help you make the necessary adjustments so that you can be successful.

Your Role in CBT for OCD

The association between interpersonal factors and the outcome of CBT is clear: the more family accommodation and hostility are involved, the weaker the effects of CBT. That's the case regardless of whether the person with OCD is an adult or a child. Yet we also know reducing accommodation and promoting healthy communication leads to a better response. So it only makes sense to include you in your loved one's CBT. That's why many therapists who work with children, or even with adults living with their parents, involve one or both parents in treatment sessions. Likewise, it makes sense to include you if the person with OCD is your intimate partner. In other instances, treatment might involve multiple family members.

Chapter 15 lays out the nuts and bolts of how you might be involved should your relative decide to seek professional treatment. My main goal in this book, however, is to help you disentangle yourself from OCD and support your relative even if your relative is *not* in therapy. As I said in the Introduction, my focus is on helping you change your own behavior with regard to your relative's OCD. Yet because the skills I'll prepare you to use in Part II, and help you apply in Part III, closely parallel CBT, it's useful to know up front what your role would be. So, here's an overview:

Learning Supportive Communication

As you'll read in detail in Chapter 9, effective communication skills are a must when the goal is to end accommodation to start breaking the vicious cycle of OCD. First and foremost, it's essential to show your love and support for your relative to preserve (or repair) family relationships and lessen conflict. But it's also important to be assertive and firm about the changes you're going to make and to stick to your plan once it's in motion. You'll learn how to clearly communicate expectations and give your loved one appropriate space to be successful on her own. Likewise, you'll learn how to use praise and rewards appropriately and how to be firm in withholding such incentives when they have not been earned. Of course, the style of communication you'll use will depend on your loved one's age and his relationship to you.

Assisting with ERP

Doing ERP is hard work, but research shows that receiving encouragement and emotional support during treatment dramatically increases its short- and long-term effects. Therefore, you'll learn how to be an effective coach and cheerleader for your relative, helping him plan and implement exposure practices and encouraging him to *work through* the obsessional anxiety. You'll also help him resist urges to ritualize as opposed to trying to alleviate the distress for him. Coaching a loved one through ERP can be challenging. After all, it's uncomfortable watching someone you love experience anxiety when you know you're not supposed to step in to make everything better. And perhaps you're someone who tends to avoid anxiety as well. Chapter 15 of this book, however, will prepare you for success.

Reducing Accommodation

If your relative decides to get professional help, the therapist will work with you to support her progress by developing a plan to reduce any accommodation you're currently providing. Because reducing accommodation is mainly dependent on how you respond to your family member's OCD, you can get started any time and don't have to wait for her to agree to enter treatment. In fact, the centerpiece of this book is a program, presented in Parts II and III, for supporting your loved one by reducing accommodation *whether or not your family member is getting professional help*. As you'll read in Chapter 5, your loved one might not be ready to seek therapy when you want her to— and you can't force her into treatment. But that doesn't have to stop *you* from beginning the process of reducing your (and others') involvement in her OCD symptoms and working toward a more functional environment for your family.

PART II

Preparing to Untangle Yourself from OCD

5

Why Your Loved One
May Refuse Treatment—
and What You Can Do

'll never forget the day I received a desperate call from Eduardo's father:

> "I think my 17-year-old son has symptoms of OCD, but no matter what we do he won't go for help. He gets anxious and angry if we even try to talk to him about it. My wife thinks we should do whatever it takes to keep him calm. But things are getting worse. He makes the whole family obey his ridiculous rules about cleanliness, or else he gets very angry and threatens us. There are arguments every day. I'm basically a hostage in my own home. You have no idea how frustrating this is. How can we make him agree to get treatment?"

I made it clear to Eduardo's father that I felt terrible about his situation and understood his frustration. And then I explained that, sadly, if Eduardo was so adamantly opposed to treatment, there would be little I could do to change him. After all, ERP is hard work even when the person is eager and fully on board. Instead, I invited Mom and Dad to make an appointment to speak with me (without Eduardo) about what *they* might do to change how *they* interacted with their son around OCD. I proposed that rather than "How can we make him agree to get treatment?," the important question was "How can we, as parents, stand by our principles without being drawn into arguing or going along with OCD?" Indeed, regardless of whether Eduardo was ready to cooperate, it would be up to his parents to make changes at home to teach Eduardo that (1) he is capable of managing his emotions and OCD symptoms in healthier ways and (2) it's worthwhile for him to do so.

Things for Ariel were a little different. On her own, she'd often thought about getting help for OCD and even had a stash of referral information and self-help books. Occasionally she'd look through this material, thinking how nice it would be to put all this in the rearview mirror. No more obsessing about danger. No more wasting time checking and rechecking. Best of all, it would make Ben happy and improve their marriage. But on the other hand, ERP treatment sounded very scary. It would be hard to give up the checking rituals. And wouldn't this put her family at risk of a burglary or fire? So in the end, she would talk herself out of getting help: "As bad as it is to have OCD, doing ERP would be even worse," she would conclude. Besides, Ariel knew when the going got tough she could somehow talk Ben into helping with checking rituals. As a result, nothing changed.

Do these stories sound familiar? I unfortunately get phone calls from people like Eduardo's father on a regular basis. A child with obsessional fears of causing bad luck refuses to do homework involving exposure to the number 13. An adult daughter still lives at home and doesn't want to admit that she's got a real problem. Similarly, I get calls from partners and spouses of people like Ariel who can't quite bring themselves to seek treatment. Maybe it's the fear of doing ERP that keeps them away—or perhaps there are other factors. In this chapter, you'll learn about the reasons your loved one with OCD might reject professional help. You'll also learn about changes you can make that will help you untangle yourself from OCD and at the same time help your loved one become more confident and independent—regardless of whether she decides to get help. Let's begin with what it's like for your loved one as she considers the prospect of treatment.

Readiness for Change and Ambivalence

As you've read, ERP isn't just "talk therapy." It requires active participation and the willpower to confront anxiety-provoking situations while resisting the urge to do anxiety-reducing rituals. So, you shouldn't be surprised if your relative is less than enthusiastic about this process. Maybe your teenager is ashamed of the content of his obsessional thoughts about sex and doesn't want to disclose them. Perhaps your partner is so terrified of becoming ill that she can't imagine doing exposure to feared contaminants. Many people with

OCD rely heavily on others' "help" with avoidance and rituals and don't want to let go of this accommodation because it feels like it's working for them. If your loved one has agreed to get treatment, these factors certainly affect how much she improves. But they might also be preventing your relative from starting treatment in the first place.

Five Stages of Change

Psychologists James Prochaska and Carlo DiClemente have identified five stages people go through as they decide whether to change something about themselves (and how hard to work at making changes). I've summarized these stages in the box below. People who are refusing treatment are likely at one of the initial stages, the first of which is *precontemplation*. This stage is typified by having no intent whatsoever to seek help for OCD. Eduardo avoids any discussion related to the topic and likely doesn't consider OCD a big enough problem to invest the time and energy for successful treatment. If your loved one is in the second stage, *contemplation,* then, like Ariel, she's bothered by having OCD and can see the benefits of changing. But she's also mindful of how much work it will take and how scary it might be to make these changes—and that's what usually leads to putting off getting started . . . if she starts at all.

I need to be honest here: you've got your work cut out for you if your

---

Which Stage of Change Characterizes Your Loved One with OCD?

Stage	Description
Precontemplation	Shows no interest in getting help and avoids any discussion of the topic
Contemplation	Sees both the pros and cons of treatment but still avoids it
Preparation	Leans toward getting help and might have even started the process
Action	Has started treatment on her own
Maintenance	Has made clear progress in treatment

loved one is at either of these first two stages, especially if she's an adult. But don't panic, and certainly don't try to use coercion or intimidation to get her into treatment against her will—a mistake many frustrated family members make. Resorting to threats ("We'll kick you out of the house if you don't go to therapy"), guilt trips ("How can you do this to me after all the love I've shown you?"), or deception ("I didn't tell her we were going to a therapist") will backfire in the end. These tactics will only make your relative leery of the process of therapy and mistrustful of you. Instead, you'll need a healthy dose of patience and perseverance. Fortunately, the techniques I'll teach you can help. I've seen them nudge people just enough that they decide to seek treatment. Perhaps more important, regardless of your relative's decision about getting help, *you'll* learn how to become disentangled from your relative's OCD symptoms—thoughtfully, compassionately, and without a guilty conscience—so you can promote healthy living for yourself and your family.

Has your loved one made calls to treatment providers on his own (or asked you to do so if he's a child) or even scheduled an appointment? If so, and if he seriously intends to begin treatment, he's at the *preparation* stage. And if he's actually begun doing ERP or started a medication, he's at the *action* stage. Finally, if your relative has already made noticeable progress in overcoming OCD, he's at the *maintenance* stage. Consider yourself fortunate if your relative is at one of these three stages of change. You can use the techniques in this book to provide the kind of coaching and cheerleading that will keep him (and your family) on the road to getting over OCD for good.

Mixed Feelings: Ambivalence

Even if on the outside your relative seems dead set against treatment, you can rest assured that on the inside he's got mixed thoughts and feelings. Your son would rather be done with obsessional fears so he can feel better about himself. Your daughter doesn't want to go on hiding her embarrassing bathroom rituals from her peers any longer. Your spouse is tired of the ongoing arguments over OCD and afraid it will affect the kids. These kinds of mixed emotions about treatment are normal. We call them *ambivalence*—the state of having opposing positive and negative feelings at the same time. Maybe your relative is totally fed up with how his religious obsessions are ruining his life, yet he's also afraid treatment would turn him into an atheist. Eduardo didn't really like being stuck in his room or having to do compulsive washing rituals, but he also thought these strategies were necessary to avoid illnesses. The thing about ambivalence is that it doesn't push your loved one to take any action. At best, he'll stay "on the fence." At worst, he's made the decision (at least for now) to refuse any help. Neither is a good option because it maintains the status quo of continuing to struggle with OCD.

Why Does Your Loved One Refuse Treatment?

The simple answer is that your loved one refuses treatment because his reasons for refusing it outweigh his reasons for pursuing it. I don't mean to be snarky—it's just a matter of *incentives.* Incentives are what push us to put effort into something. They're the answer to the question "What's in it for me?" Money, for instance, is an incentive because it gets people to go to work. The prospect of getting lung cancer (as well as the cost of a pack of cigarettes) is an incentive to quit smoking. Getting help for OCD works the same way. The decision to invest the time and effort, and endure the discomfort of doing a treatment like ERP requires that your relative have plenty of good reasons (incentives) for doing so and relatively few reasons for not doing so.

Don't confuse incentives with *motivation,* which is more like *wanting* something. Your loved one probably *wants* to be done with OCD. But wanting something is not the same as working hard for it. You might *want* to learn how to play the guitar, yet without the necessary incentive to put the effort into finding a teacher, going to lessons, and spending time practicing, you won't reach your goal. So, if your loved one is refusing treatment for OCD, it means she lacks the incentive necessary to take action—not necessarily the desire to get better. Maybe doing ERP and confronting fear triggers seems too scary or overwhelming. Maybe she doesn't fully appreciate the negative consequences of having OCD or realize how much better her life and relationships could be without this disorder. Here are the most important factors that reduce your relative's incentive to engage in treatment.

Fear of ERP

If you've ever found yourself face to face with something you were afraid of, you can appreciate why your relative might feel skittish about the prospect of doing ERP. After all, she puts a great deal of time and effort into *avoiding* the very same fearful situations and stimuli she'd have to face head-on as part of treatment. This, along with giving up her rituals, might seem like too much of a risk to take. Your loved one might also be afraid of experiencing "too much" fear during exposure. Naturally, to at least some extent, the perception that ERP will be too difficult or anxiety provoking can reduce the incentive to engage in this treatment for people of all ages with OCD.

Negative Attitudes about Medication

Negative beliefs about psychiatric medications are also common. Your loved one might perceive herself as stigmatized, emotionally weak, or unable to manage her problems if she has to go on one of these drugs. Perhaps she's tried them before but found them unhelpful. In addition, unfavorable news reports and ethical scandals have left the pharmaceutical industry with a black eye and led many would-be consumers away from these products. Your loved one might also be wary of side effects or opposed to chemically altering her brain. All of these concerns reduce the incentive to take medications for OCD.

Poor Insight

Your loved one might feel very strongly that her obsessions are realistic and her rituals are worthwhile—what clinicians call "poor insight." For instance, it made perfect sense to Ariel to be absolutely certain the doors were locked and the appliances off before she left the house or went to bed. To her, the extensive checking rituals kept her family out of harm's way. After all, there had never been any break-ins or fires as long as she'd been checking! Ariel's rituals also helped her control obsessional fear, even though they provided only short-term relief and maintained the problem in the long run. Nevertheless, to Ariel the rituals appeared to work, which made them difficult to surrender. Ariel didn't want to try ERP because she knew that agreeing to treatment would mean having to give up her rituals.

Fear of Getting Better

Believe it or not, your loved one might refuse treatment because there's a part of him that feels threatened by getting rid of OCD. This is especially likely if he's had OCD for a long time or his symptoms have resulted in substantial functional impairment. After being immersed in obsessions and rituals for years on end, he might have become used to feeling anxious and engaging in compulsive behaviors. Maybe he's accepted not working, not going to school, and not having much of a social life as "familiar" and "normal." Although difficult for you to understand, the prospect of being free of OCD might seem foreign or scary to your relative since it involves a new and unfamiliar set of feelings, thoughts, and behaviors.

And let's not forget new and unfamiliar *expectations,* which can seem especially threatening. Xavier, who had lived with his parents for many years, was afraid that if his OCD got better, his parents would demand more of him. He'd be given more responsibilities, expected to live on his own, go back to work full-time, push himself socially, and the like. Your loved one might be wary of these and other responsibilities, such as having to succeed in school, help with chores around the house, and maintain general health and cleanliness. It's as if continuing to live with OCD (and avoiding increased expectations) is the lesser of two evils.

Hopelessness, Helplessness, and Depression

Your loved one might believe that he can't be helped and that life without obsessions and rituals sounds too good to be true. Maybe your son or daughter thinks recovery from OCD is impossible to achieve, so there's no point in even trying. Perhaps your spouse or partner has previously attempted therapy—ERP or otherwise—without much success and feels discouraged about trying again. It's not hard to understand how feeling this way reduces the incentive to put in the hard work necessary for helping oneself get over OCD.

Symptom Accommodation

Under most circumstances the natural consequences of having OCD—emotional distress, inconvenience, and embarrassment—are strong incentives for pursuing treatment. But, as you've already learned, accommodation protects your relative from bearing the full brunt of the problem. Eduardo's mother, for example, worked so hard to accommodate Eduardo's obsessions and compulsions that she actually ended up suffering more from his problem than he did. Maybe it doesn't sound so terrible to help a loved one so that his life is less painful—except that a little "help" almost always leads to getting pulled into doing more. And the more accommodation you offer, the easier you make it for your relative to live with OCD and the less incentive he has to do the hard work on his own to get better.

I know discontinuing accommodation sounds difficult—and you've probably got your own mixed thoughts and feelings (ambivalence) about whether and how much to pull back. In the chapters that follow, however, I'll prepare you to skillfully reduce accommodation so that your relative's distress becomes an incentive to get help and put OCD behind her (this is sometimes referred to as "tough love"). The three chapters in Part II (including this one) lay an important foundation for discontinuing accommodation and supporting your relative in other ways; in Part III you'll learn how to stop accommodating OCD step by step.

Denial

Another way families or intimate partners inadvertently contribute to treatment refusal is by denying or minimizing the severity of OCD symptoms. Nicholas knew Linda was extremely embarrassed by her obsessional thoughts and avoidance, so he swept them under the rug even though he knew it was something that needed to be discussed and dealt with. Maybe *you* look the other way when your child is stuck doing rituals. Maybe you explain away your spouse's extreme avoidance behavior as just "quirky." Talking about these issues can be uncomfortable—for you and for your loved one. You might wonder if it's even worth bringing them up. Yet the message that *not* raising these issues sends is "We don't need to deal with obsessions and rituals," and this may lead your relative further away from treatment. Sure, you don't want to be overly harsh or critical, but there *is* a healthy middle ground.

Conflict and Hostility

Do your homework! Put your clothes in the hamper! Go to bed! Your young child has lots of experience resisting parental demands that she views as imposing on her autonomy. Your adult child or intimate partner can be just as resentful (*Pick up the kids from school! Take out the trash! Put down the toilet seat!*). Maybe things have become so hostile that, out of spite, your loved one is simply motivated to defy your wish that she get help for OCD. Communication patterns such as nagging, yelling, making threats, or shaming only make things worse by sending the message that you think your loved one can just change his behavior because of something you (or other family members) *say*. Advice about communicating effectively is presented in Chapter 7, but for now, know that these negative interactions don't provide an incentive to get treatment and only lead to more conflict.

So What Can You Do?

It sure seems like knowledge and awareness should be enough to convince your relative to do something about OCD. If not, then using threats and punishment should do the trick, right? Unfortunately, it doesn't work that way. But your past attempts to get your loved one to go for help have failed *not* because your lectures, sermons, and threats weren't convincing enough, but because you simply can't make someone change who's not ready. In other words, it's your *agenda* of trying to lecture or arm-wrestle your relative into going to treatment that's the problem. It simply can't work.

That's why I'm suggesting a different agenda—one you have complete control over. This agenda involves focusing entirely on making changes to *your own* approach. As hard as it is to accept, your relative has the right to refuse treatment. But when you focus on changing your own frame of mind and your own behavior when it comes to OCD, you'll be in a much better position to respond supportively by resisting demands for help with avoidance, rituals, and other accommodation. This means that instead of working on reducing your loved one's OCD symptoms (something that is best left to a qualified mental health professional), you'll be working to minimize the negative effects that these symptoms currently have in your household.

Although the changes I'll help you make are in your loved one's best interests and will not harm him, it's only normal for there to be an adjustment period (for which I will prepare you). But sticking with this program is the best way to support your loved one and improve your (and your family's) quality of life, even if your loved one decides not to step up to the plate himself. And who knows? Your changes might lead him to decide that it's worthwhile to join forces with you or seek professional help on his own.

Believe it or not, your new agenda begins with making sure you're taking care of yourself and managing your own stress, so read on.

Taking Care of Yourself

You've probably noticed when you fly on an airplane that the flight attendant always instructs you to put on *your* oxygen mask before helping others. Why? Because if *you* run out of oxygen, you can't help anyone else! In a similar vein, if you don't take good care of yourself and prioritize your own needs once in a while, you simply won't have the physical and mental stamina to do what's necessary to support your relative and improve things in your household.

Giving Yourself Permission

When I suggested that Xavier's parents leave Xavier at home and take that vacation they'd been talking about for several years, they gave me strange looks: "Isn't that selfish!? How can we pamper ourselves when our son's suffering with so much anxiety?" And when I advised Ben to join a bowling league with his friends—which Ariel was dead set against—he was concerned about leaving his wife home alone with their kids: "That's going to make her very angry, and things will be even worse!" Do you have similar concerns that deter you from attending to your own well-being? If so, they can be very persuasive and powerful. But these concerns are simply not justified. Let's look at them more carefully.

Is it selfish to look out for yourself? Your partner, spouse, or child is struggling with OCD, so how could you possibly put *your own* needs first? But taking care of yourself isn't a luxury; it's a *necessity*. Think of your body as a car. With the right fuel and proper maintenance, it will run reliably. But neglect its upkeep, and it will start to give you trouble. Just like wear and tear on a car, caregiver stress is real. And you've got to be at the top of your game both physically and mentally if you're going to support your loved one and make your home environment more pleasant. So, if you neglect your own maintenance, it's going to catch up with you sooner or later. The long and short of it is that by concentrating on your own well-being you're actually nurturing the most valuable asset your loved one has—*you*—and that's anything but selfish.

Will your relative be upset? Of course she will! Your loved one's going to be upset with any changes to the usual routine. Ariel was pretty mad when Ben informed her that he was joining the bowling league and would be out every Monday night with his friends. But remember one of the guiding principles of this book: you can control only your own behavior—not your relative's. So, it's really up to *her* if she gets upset. Moreover, this kind of distress is temporary and harmless (as you'll learn in the next chapter). And if her anger is a reminder that OCD is keeping her from feeling more at ease and doing more things she'd like to do, then it's actually an incentive to change. Also, keep in mind that there's no guarantee your relative *won't* get upset even if you *don't* change your behavior. So, whether or not she gets upset doesn't have much to do with the choices you make. The choice you have is whether or not to improve your own quality of life.

Do you need to be there for your relative all the time? Eduardo's mother had quit her job so she could stay home with Eduardo full-time. But she was quickly becoming frustrated and burned out being in the house all the time and dealing with Eduardo's OCD-driven demands. I suggested she'd benefit from taking a break each day and getting out of the house—maybe a long walk or joining a gym and exercising. Yet as much as she wanted a break from OCD, she felt guilty about taking "me time": "There's no time for a break. Eduardo can't be alone. If I go out, he'll get anxious and there will be no one to calm him down." But Eduardo didn't *need* his mother present. Staying home was merely an unnecessary accommodation behavior that (ironically) prevented him from learning to manage anxiety on his own. (I'll help you understand why this is true in the next chapter.) Second, Eduardo's mother was overlooking the fact that taking some daily "me time" would help recharge her battery and reduce the unwanted feelings of frustration and guilt. She'd be more level-headed and able to use constructive strategies to manage things with her son.

Changing Unhealthy Thinking Patterns to Reduce Stress

Our thoughts and attitudes play an important role in determining our feelings and behaviors. So if you frequently find yourself feeling depressed, anxious, angry, or guilty over situations involving your relative and OCD, it's worth looking carefully at what you're *telling yourself* about the situation. You're likely to find exaggerated and self-defeating ideas and beliefs. Fortunately, becoming more aware of these kinds of thinking patterns, and then challenging yourself to examine all sides of the issue and get a more accurate perspective, will help you control your stress levels. I'm not suggesting you simply "think positively." Rather, the key is to think more *rationally*. Let's take a look at some common stress-inducing thinking patterns, as well as how to defuse them.

Overgeneralizing

When you take something you don't like about a person or a situation (for example, Ariel not wanting Ben to go bowling) and you exaggerate it until it seems like a never-ending pattern (Ariel *never* lets me do *anything* with my friends), you're overgeneralizing. Other examples include "He *always* uses his OCD as an excuse" and "*Everyone* else's family is normal." This thinking pattern leads to a build-up of irritation and hopelessness. What's worse, you just end up looking for evidence to confirm your overgeneralization, so things seem worse than they really are. If you carefully examine your overgeneralizations, you'll see that they're probably oversimplified and inaccurate.

Reduce your tendency to overgeneralize by looking for words like *always, never, everyone,* and *no one*. Since they're rarely true, throw them out and replace them with more flexible words like *sometimes, some people,* and *usually*. Also, try to stick to the facts and notice situations that prove your overgeneralization wrong—for example, the fun activities you share with your loved one or that day he took a normal shower and got to school on time. Finally, ask yourself if you're using *all-or-nothing thinking,* an extreme form of overgeneralization in which you see anything short of perfection as a total failure. Instead, try to see the middle ground, such as "he is successful at some things, but not at others." These strategies can help you soften your attachment to overgeneralizations and put you in a better frame of mind for supporting your relative with OCD.

Fortune Telling

Sometimes we think like fortune-tellers or psychics, believing we can see into the future and assuming things will turn out badly before they even happen. Do you jump right to the worst-case scenario and tell yourself things like "I just know his OCD is going to ruin our vacation" or "You'll see—she's going to fail out of school"? Perhaps you've already decided that your loved one will never get better and that the difficulties you're facing will last forever. Maybe you jump to the conclusion that your relative is on the verge of a nervous breakdown from all of her anxiety. Finally, there's *mind reading,* a form of fortune telling where you believe you know what other people are thinking without any facts to back up your belief (for example, "The neighbors will think we're bad parents if they find out about our daughter's OCD").

If you notice yourself fortune telling, try asking yourself what the evidence is to support the conclusions you're jumping to and what the evidence is against your conclusions. When you look at the facts, you'll probably find the dreaded outcome is less likely than you've anticipated. Also, you *don't* have a crystal ball. So remind yourself that your assumptions are only guesses. Have there been similar situations in the past when you expected something bad to happen, only to have your prediction not come true? How might someone else look at the situation, or what would you say to a friend who was in the same circumstances? Finally, try reminding yourself that *feeling* anxious and stressed out doesn't automatically mean your worries are realistic. Thinking through these questions might not completely alleviate your stress, but they'll help you get a more realistic perspective so you're only as anxious as the facts warrant.

Musts and Shoulds

In this thinking pattern you've convinced yourself that you or others *must* or *should* behave the way you expect (for example, "I *must* make sure he never becomes anxious," "She *should* go to therapy," or "He *shouldn't* argue with me"). The problem here is that you've set overly rigid and unrealistic expectations. If you place such demands on yourself, you'll feel guilty when you inevitably fall short of your mandate. And if the *should*s are directed at someone else, you'll feel anger and resentment when at some point that person fails to follow your rules.

To curb this thinking pattern, try swapping out the *should*s and *must*s for more flexible and realistic thinking, such as "I *wish* my son didn't have to go through so much anxiety" and "It would sure be *easier* if she'd get help." I'm not saying to just give up on making things better—far from it. But if you remember that reality is complex, and things happen independently of our wishes, you'll experience less frustration and stress and be in a better position to effectively support your loved one.

"I Can't Stand It" Thinking

When you tell yourself that you "can't stand it," you take setbacks, annoyances, and inconveniences and needlessly turn them into unbearable catastrophes, leading to unnecessary and counterproductive reactions like rage, dread, and horror. But even if in that moment you feel that you really can't stand the situation, the truth is you *can* stand it. How do I know? Because if you're reading this, you've survived 100% of the time!

Let's be clear: some situations are legitimately upsetting, and I'm not saying you need to feel *positive* about them. But that doesn't mean you can't *tolerate* them. The next time you find yourself thinking that you "can't stand it," consider whether you've dealt with a similar situation in the past. If so, you've just proven that you *are* capable of handling it. In fact, is there really any situation that you literally can't stand? Besides being fatally wounded or deprived of oxygen, food, and water—which are vital for staying alive—you can stand just about *anything*.

Labeling

Labeling means taking one behavior or characteristic of a person and using it as an overall characterization. Because your son is afraid of knives, he's a "wuss." Because your wife won't get help for OCD, she's "lazy." Your daughter cursed at you, so she's "rotten." But the problem is that people can't be reduced to one label—we're much too complex. So your son isn't a "wuss"; he has obsessional fears of knives. Your wife isn't "lazy"; there might not be enough incentive for her to decide it's worth seeking help. Your daughter isn't "rotten"; she said some curse words.

Labeling makes you feel miserable about your loved one (or yourself). So when you catch yourself falling into this trap, try describing the behavior you don't like instead: "He's doing a ritual"; "She's avoiding getting help"; "She cursed at me." Sure, you don't like these behaviors (and it may well be worth working toward changing them), but remember that everyone has strengths and weaknesses, and we all make mistakes sometimes.

6

Learning the Facts
about Anxiety, Obsessions,
and Uncertainty

Many people I work with find it challenging to push themselves and their loved ones. From my experience with many couples and families affected by OCD, it's clear that a major obstacle to reducing accommodation is the fear that this kind of "tough love" will cause harm—either physically or emotionally. Maybe you worry that if you stop doing rituals for your husband, he will become so anxious that he has a breakdown; or that your daughter's bizarre obsessional thoughts will cause her to lose control unless you do something to stop them. How can you be expected to reduce your involvement in OCD if you're concerned about such things?

Fortunately concerns like these are based on misunderstandings about anxiety, obsessions, and the experience of uncertainty—all of which are actually safe. In fact, ERP works by helping people "lean into" these experiences over and over so they can learn that they're not harmful. My aim in this chapter, therefore, is to give you the facts so that you're able to feel more confident about reducing accommodation when the time comes to do so.

Understanding Anxiety

When Xavier refused to get help for his OCD, his parents wisely stopped trying to twist his arm and instead sought help on their own (without Xavier). But the minute the therapist suggested Mom and Dad begin cutting back on all the accommodation they were doing, there was a firm objection. "We know we're enabling Xavier," they said, "but you don't realize how harmful it is for him to have so much anxiety. With his OCD, he's been through so much, and we don't know if his nerves can take much more. He doesn't eat or sleep when he's anxious, and we don't want him to go over the edge." Xavier's parents wanted to help their son, but how could they stop accommodating his OCD when they believed anxiety would harm him?

Ariel often played the "anxiety card" to get Ben to help with her checking rituals: "I'm having a panic attack because I can't remember if I unplugged my hair dryer this morning!" she would frantically exclaim over the phone. "I can't catch my breath . . . I feel faint and lightheaded . . . I can't take this much longer. You have to go home and check for me. . . . Please, Ben, it's the only thing that will make this awful feeling go away . . . *please!*" The way Ariel described her anxious feelings scared Ben. To him, she was vulnerable—like a flickering candle flame that needed to be shielded from the wind. So he routinely gave in even though it meant driving 30 minutes home and 30 minutes back to work in the middle of the day.

Do you have similar concerns that anxiety will harm your relative? If so, these concerns might keep you from successfully reducing accommodation. The good news, though, is that anxiety won't harm your family member. People with OCD are not like fragile, flickering candle flames—so you don't need to create a "no wind zone." Nor do you have to worry about your relative *going over the edge* from too much anxiety or distress. *There is no edge.* But anxiety is complex, so understanding exactly what's happening to your loved one when she's anxious is an important step in feeling more confident disconnecting from her OCD.

I introduced the idea that anxiety is really hard to ignore in Chapter 2, because this is a fundamental part of the nature of OCD. The fight-or-flight response is hardwired in all of us, and that's why your relative's obsessional fear and anxiety are no different from the anxiety *you* feel from time to time. As explained earlier, anxiety might come up more often and more intensely for your relative, but it still is not, in and of itself, harmful.

What Will Anxiety Do to My Loved One?

The worst thing anxiety will do is make your relative feel afraid. But because the physical effects and feelings of apprehension can be intense and unpleasant, they can *seem* like something terrible: imminent death, fainting, insanity, or some other terrible loss of control. So it's helpful to know the facts about what anxiety can, and can't, do to your loved one.

One of the most alarming physical sensations associated with anxiety is an increase in heart rate and the strength of the heartbeat. Yet as scary as this feels, it's necessary for survival if, say, you're trying not to become some wild animal's dinner. The heart pumps blood, which carries oxygen (and other nutrients) to the muscles and other tissues. Muscles use oxygen and nutrients for energy, and the racing or pounding heart during periods of high anxiety keeps it coming. Likewise, breathing automatically becomes faster and deeper. This ensures that blood pumping through the body is rich with oxygen to fuel any activity that might be needed to escape or fight off danger. Sometimes this can cause the harmless (but frightening) sensation that you're choking, suffocating, or can't catch your breath. It also causes fluctuations in levels of oxygen (an increase) and carbon dioxide (a decrease) in the bloodstream, which can lead to feelings of faintness or dizziness, blurred vision, confusion, feelings of unreality (as if you are in a dream), and hot flashes. But although these sensations are uncomfortable, they're temporary and completely benign, disappearing once breathing returns to typical levels.

Digesting food also requires a lot of energy, but when danger is perceived, the primary goal is survival (you can "rest and digest" once you're out of harm's way). Therefore, the digestive system temporarily slows down so the body can conserve energy and redirect it to the muscles needed for fight or flight. This can cause nausea, heavy feelings in your stomach, and diarrhea. There is also a decrease in appetite—fight-or-flight is not the time to stop and eat.

When a threat is perceived and anxiety is triggered, the brain goes on high alert, scanning its surroundings and analyzing the situation to look for signs of danger. This is useful when there's an actual threat to prepare for. But when it's just a false alarm—as is the case with OCD—it leads to obsessional preoccupation, feelings of apprehension, and trouble focusing, remembering, or concentrating on other things. Your loved one might also have trouble sleeping when he's anxious. Of course, none of this means there is anything wrong with your relative's brain. It's simply doing what it's supposed to do when it encounters a perceived threat (falling asleep when danger is lurking is *not* a recipe for survival). Also, these effects are temporary, and things return to normal once the anxiety passes.

Finally, anxiety is associated with the buildup of nervous energy and the overwhelming urge to release this energy. Does your relative become angry, hostile, or even violent when anxious? Maybe she can restrain herself from acting destructively, but the aggressive urges might still sneak out in other ways, such as starting arguments or intentionally saying nasty or sarcastic things. Even nervous habits such as pacing, tapping, and nail biting are ways of releasing this energy. OCD-related avoidance and rituals are also part of this response since their purpose is to escape from perceived danger and bring about a sense of safety.

It's important to know that all of these effects are temporary. The chemical messengers that produce the fight-or-flight response (adrenaline and noradrenaline) are eventually broken down by other chemicals in the body. In other words, anxiety won't continue forever, nor spiral to ever-increasing or harmful levels.

What Will Anxiety Not Do?

Do you worry that too much anxiety will cause your relative to have a breakdown, lose control, become paralyzed, or act in strange or terrible ways? Remember that the fight-or-flight response is designed to *help* when threat is perceived. So, although it seems like he's confused or overwhelmed, he's actually able to think *faster* and react *more quickly* than he normally would. Some families worry that too much anxiety will cause their relative with OCD to have a psychotic break or develop schizophrenia—a serious mental disorder characterized by hallucinations (for example, hearing voices that aren't really there), strange delusions (such as the belief you're receiving telepathic messages from government officials), and incoherent thinking and speech. But psychosis and schizophrenia begin gradually rather than suddenly, usually run in families, and are easy for mental health professionals to recognize. If your loved one has been interviewed by a mental health expert and not been diagnosed with these problems, it's extremely unlikely she'll develop them now. Finally, there is no evidence that schizophrenia is brought on by increased anxiety.

Another common worry is that "too much" anxiety will weaken the body or cause medical problems, such as a stroke or heart condition. Yet although the dizziness and pain your loved one experiences are real, they result from the intense breathing patterns and muscle tension associated with the fight-or-flight response. Dizziness results from an abrupt increase in oxygen levels, and the headaches and chest pain are focused in the *muscles,* not the brain or heart. Those muscles only hurt because they're tired from the intense breathing. So, there's no actual threat to any vital organs. On the other hand, chronic stress over many decades does indeed increase the risk of heart disease and stroke as we age; yet this is different from the fight-or-flight response, which involves short-term bursts of adrenaline, similar in many ways to what happens during physical exercise.

I've also worked with family members who were afraid too much anxiety would cause fainting or nervous collapse, or "wear out" their loved one's nerves. But the fight-or-flight response is incompatible with fainting. The muscle *tension* that occurs is the opposite of the muscle *relaxation* that happens during fainting spells. Fainting occurs when blood pressure and heart rate *drop*; yet the fight-or-flight response *increases* heart rate and blood pressure. And even if your relative were to faint, consciousness is usually regained within a few seconds. Fainting is simply a way for the body to return to a normal level of functioning. Finally, contrary to what many people believe, nerves are not like electrical wires—no amount of anxiety can wear them out or use them up.

In summary, the purpose of the anxiety response is to *protect* us from harm. And it would make no sense for nature to develop a response to threat that leads to fatal medical conditions, a loss of control, or nervous collapse (which would have surely spelled the annihilation of our ancestors).

What Should You Do?

It's not your job to bring your loved one's anxiety to an end; anxiety is safe and manageable. If she's not willing to seek professional help to learn this through therapy, you can adjust your own attitude and behavior to help her learn this valuable lesson. Use what you've read here to help her distinguish between *danger* and *discomfort*. It's OK to feel uncomfortable and afraid—everyone does from time to time. Accept and validate her experience and let her know you're confident she can tolerate these feelings and get through the discomfort. Use it as an opportunity to help her learn that she *can* manage anxiety. When your loved one is successful, reward her triumphs with praise, a pat on the back, or perhaps something more substantial (see Chapter 10). These are valuable lessons that will help her, as well as your family, in the long run.

Demystifying Obsessional Thoughts

When Xavier was 10 years old, he was standing with his family waiting for a subway train in New York City when the thought of pushing his little sister onto the tracks in front of a speeding train went through his mind. Xavier was scared—he adored his sister and would never want to hurt her. But when he told his parents about the thought he'd had, they became alarmed and immediately hustled the family out of the subway station. Xavier's mother said, "What's the matter with you, Xavier? How could you even *think* like that? Do you want something awful to happen?" His father told Xavier to try thinking positive thoughts instead and even gave him a rubber band to put around his wrist and snap himself every time a "bad thought" came to mind. As far as Xavier's parents were concerned, these intrusive thoughts were potentially dangerous, and Xavier needed to control them more effectively.

In Chapter 2, you learned that obsessional fear develops when your loved one misinterprets senseless intrusive thoughts as highly significant and threatening. But just like Xavier's parents and many concerned family members I've worked with, maybe you're still uneasy about your loved one's obsessional thoughts. Perhaps you're not convinced they're safe and mean-ingless. Or you believe they can and should be controlled. Maybe you try to help your relative with OCD dismiss or avoid her obsessions; or you analyze them together and provide reassurance that everything is going to be OK. But if you're going to be successful in supporting your loved one while also get-ting out from under OCD, you'll need to recognize that obsessions are harm-less pieces of mental driftwood—not bloodthirsty sharks. And you'll need to respond to them accordingly so you can promote confidence in your family member's ability to manage these thoughts without accommodation. Keep-ing the following points in mind will help.

Unwanted Intrusive Thoughts Are Normal

We all have them—people with and without OCD alike. In fact, research shows that 90–99% of people around the world say that they sometimes have random, senseless, upsetting, and bizarre thoughts, even some that go against their morality, sexuality, and personality (and the 1–10% who say they don't have these kinds of thoughts are probably fibbing). And why not? Thousands of thoughts go through our mind each day, so you'd expect that some are going to be unwanted or unpleasant. Just to prove my point, I've included the box on pages 79–80, which contains a list of intrusive thoughts reported by people *without* OCD. I compiled this list with the help of a large group of friends, relatives, students, and colleagues—and even included some of my own unwanted thoughts.

Why is it normal—even beneficial—to have these kinds of thoughts? Our minds are great at imagining bad things that could happen so that we're more careful and do the right thing. If we see someone walking by the side of the road, our minds can easily imagine "What if I hit him with my car?" But having this image come to mind only helps prevent disaster by focusing us to drive more carefully.

One of the most famous studies on obsessional thoughts took place in 1978, when psychologists Jack Rachman and Padmal de Silva gave trained

Intrusive Thoughts Reported by People without OCD

HARM- OR DEATH-RELATED THOUGHTS

- Thoughts of running the car off the road or into oncoming traffic
- Thoughts of poking something into your eyes
- Thoughts of jumping (or pushing someone else) in front of an oncoming car or train
- Ideas about doing something mean or violent to a loved one or to a defenseless or undeserving person

THOUGHTS ABOUT BEING RESPONSIBLE FOR HARM OR DISASTERS

- Thoughts of causing an accident or mishap
- Thoughts of getting into an accident while driving with children in the car
- Thoughts that you've forgotten something important

THOUGHTS ABOUT CONTAMINATION

- Thoughts of having a terrible disease
- Thoughts that you may have caught a disease from touching a toilet seat
- Thoughts of dirt and germs being on your hands
- Thoughts of passing germs or illness to another person

THOUGHTS ABOUT ACTING INAPPROPRIATELY

- Ideas about insulting or abusing family or friends for no apparent reason
- Thoughts of using racial slurs to offend people
- Thoughts of swearing or screaming rudely at your family
- Impulses to push your children away

THOUGHTS ABOUT SAFETY

- Thoughts that you left a door unlocked, which will lead to a break-in
- Thoughts that you left an electrical appliance on and caused a fire
- Thoughts that your house has burned down and you've lost everything you own
- Thoughts that maybe you didn't do enough to warn someone of potential danger

THOUGHTS RELATED TO MORALITY AND RELIGION

- Thoughts of doing something morally wrong
- Unwanted blasphemous thoughts during prayers
- Wondering about whether you have committed sins or will go to hell
- Doubts about whether you're being faithful enough
- Doubts about whether you appreciate someone or something enough

THOUGHTS OF ACTING IMPULSIVELY

- Thoughts of smashing a table full of handblown glass (at a crafts market, for example)
- Thought of doing something dramatic like robbing a bank

THOUGHTS RELATED TO SEX

- Thoughts of violence during sex
- Unwanted sexual impulses toward someone you know or don't know
- Thoughts of engaging in "unnatural" or "inappropriate" sexual acts
- Images or thoughts about someone else's genitals

mental health clinicians a list of intrusive thoughts from people *without* OCD, as well as a list of actual obsessions reported by people *with* OCD. When asked to use their clinical skills to identify which thoughts came from which group of people, the therapists were unsuccessful. This study and others like it conducted worldwide have found the same thing, which means that the upsetting obsessional thoughts your relative with OCD has are the same kinds of unwanted intrusive thoughts that just about everyone else in the world experiences too.

Why Are Obsessions Repetitive?

If your relative's obsessions are just normal thoughts, then why are they so intense and repetitive? What's wrong with her that she's so preoccupied with awful ideas and images? Deep down, does she want to do something terrible?

The answer is that the more your loved one tries to control or push away her obsessional thoughts, the more repetitive and intense they become. You can see this for yourself: just try *not* to think of a pink elephant . . . what's the first thought that crossed your mind? The pink elephant, of course! It's a psychological fact that humans are bad at controlling or dismissing thoughts. We can't keep something out of our minds without thinking about it. So, when we try not to think about something (a funny-looking pink elephant or a grim obsessional thought), it starts to morph into daily, hourly, even constant thoughts. And that's part of the trap OCD sets by using your relative's mind against her. She misinterprets obsessional thoughts as dangerous and then feels the need to dismiss or control them, which makes the obsessions multiply.

So, why does your relative have obsessional thoughts all the time? What kind of person thinks that way? Someone who doesn't want to do anything wrong—that's who.

What Should You Do?

Since obsessional thoughts—even the most disturbing and uncontrollable intrusions—are nothing more than a series of neurons firing in the brain, you don't need to be worried about their content, frequency, meaning, or intensity. Nor do you need to shield your relative from them. In fact, it's important for her to learn how to accept these thoughts as a normal part of life so she develops greater confidence in herself and reduces her dependence on others when such thoughts show up.

With this in mind, you'll want to respond in ways that deflate the significance of obsessions and treat them as normal, safe, and manageable. This means remaining calm when your relative tells you about unwanted thoughts. Validate her experience (sure, no one likes these kinds of thoughts) but highlight the difference between thoughts and actions (for example, "That sounds upsetting. It's a good thing that's just a *thought*. I have upsetting thoughts like that too, sometimes"). Then send the message that you're certain she's able to cope with and tolerate the obsession. You can suggest getting back to whatever she was doing when the thought came up. In later chapters, you'll learn the nuts and bolts of how to compassionately reduce your involvement in avoidance, rituals, giving reassurance, and other forms of accommodation in response to obsessions.

Accepting Uncertainty

Eduardo couldn't actually *see* the "bathroom germs" he was afraid of; and it was this sense of uncertainty that prompted his excessive avoidance and compulsive washing rituals just to be *extra sure* he wasn't contaminated. He'd even convinced his mother that he needed an iron clad guarantee of safety, and Mom obeyed Eduardo's rules because she wanted him to feel totally reassured. Ben also believed it was important to keep Ariel feeling *completely sure* that the doors were locked and appliances were safely turned off. That's what motivated him to drop everything and help with her rituals. "I love Ariel. How could I let her suffer with uncertainty when it's easier just to reassure her?" he thought to himself. And this usually put Ariel at ease . . . at least until the next obsession showed up.

It seemed logical to Xavier's parents to reassure their son that he *is* a morally upstanding person. Xavier's pastor addressed the problem similarly, frequently reviewing with Xavier scriptural passages and other inspired writings to guarantee Xavier that he didn't have to worry about his spiritual path. And it was similar for Nicholas, who just couldn't understand why Linda would worry about molesting their granddaughter. After all, Linda was the most kind, thoughtful, proper, and ethical person he knew. So Nicholas would try reassuring her that she loved Emma, had never harmed anyone in her life, and had never had any sexual fantasies about children or babies. Yet nothing he said seemed to take away the fact that there was still a *chance* Linda *could* do the unthinkable. Both Nicholas and Linda were frustrated.

Just like Eduardo's mother and Ariel's husband, maybe you don't like seeing your relative struggle with uncertainty. And maybe you believe it's important to comfort your loved one with reassurance. Like Xavier's parents and Linda's husband, maybe you believe that if you just keep working at it, you'll eventually convince your family member that she doesn't need to be so afraid. To get out of OCD's hold, however, you'll need to fine-tune the way you think about and respond to this kind of uncertainty. Keeping the following in mind will help.

Certainty Is an Illusion

In his book *Freedom from Obsessive–Compulsive Disorder,* Dr. Jonathan Grayson highlights the illusive nature of certainty by asking readers to think of someone they love who is not presently in the room. Try this yourself— maybe even think of your loved one with OCD (if she is not with you). Then ask yourself, "Is this person alive right now?"

Your first inclination was probably to think "Yes, of course." Maybe you just saw her or spoke with her; or maybe he's asleep down the hall. But even so, isn't it *possible* that something terrible has happened? An accident? A murder? A medical catastrophe? Maybe even within the last few minutes? And yet you're probably still feeling confident your loved one is alive even knowing this feeling is based on probability rather than absolute truth. You probably also don't have to check on the person to reassure yourself she's alive. That's because you're managing the uncertainty of this situation in a healthy way: you assume your sense of certainty is accurate and you act accordingly unless you have good reasons to indicate otherwise—such as a text, phone call, or physical evidence informing you otherwise.

Your relative's world is no more or no less uncertain than yours, yet she deals with uncertainty by focusing on the *possibilities* rather than on the *probabilities*. She believes that she can't carry on unless the uncertainty has been eliminated. What's more, she mistakenly believes it's possible to eliminate it. This is what triggers the unrelenting quest for reassurance. It's often where I see people like you getting drawn into OCD.

But your relative probably doesn't demand reassurance in *every* domain of her life. Linda had no problem with driving and even used her smartphone while on the road. Xavier liked hunting, owned a rifle, and never worried about gun accidents. Similarly, it's only where your family member's obsessional fears are concerned that she insists on certainty. In other spheres of living she's probably able to take certainty for granted just like you do (perhaps even more so). And this proves that your loved one *is* capable of managing uncertainty. Just imagine if Linda could assume she won't molest Emma the same way she assumes she can drive safely while talking on her phone. Suppose Xavier could have faith that God loves him the same way he has faith in his ability to handle firearms.

Reassurance Doesn't Work

For all of the avoidance and rituals your relative with OCD goes through, and after all the reassurance you give her, she still won't have a guarantee that what she's afraid of won't come true. Germs are microscopic, people make mistakes sometimes, religious and spiritual faith requires believing what you can't see, and no one can predict the future with certainty—people sometimes act in ways we wouldn't expect them to. Trying to reassure your family member only tightens OCD's hold because every attempt to provide reassurance legitimizes the obsession. After all, why go to such lengths to provide reassurance if there is nothing to worry about? It also strengthens the idea that uncertainty is unmanageable and that avoidance and rituals are the only way to deal with it. Finally, as you know, family members who are vital sources of support become annoyed and withdraw from the person with OCD, which only serves to raise stress levels for all parties.

What Should You Do?

If you're going to successfully abstain from providing reassurance, you'll need to keep in mind that your loved one is better at managing uncertainty than you think—*and better than she thinks*. She probably accepts uncertainty in many areas of her life that are not affected by OCD. Random acts of violence or terror and tragedies are rare, but they absolutely can and do happen. The risk isn't any greater for your relative than for anyone else. In fact, *you're* also uncertain about the situations your relative obsesses about. We all are. So acknowledge that uncertainty and doubt can feel uncomfortable and let her know that based on how well she handles uncertainty in other areas of life, you're confident she can also manage without reassurance when it comes to her obsessions. In later chapters I'll show you how to shrink your role in providing reassurance in a supportive and compassionate way that helps loosen OCD's grip on you and your family.

7

Learning
to Communicate Effectively

Eduardo's mother and father weren't on the same page when it came to dealing with OCD. His mother usually gave in and accommodated the symptoms, while his father believed OCD was just a ploy to get more attention. He'd often become frustrated and yell at his son, "What's wrong with you? You're old enough to clean your own damn room. And what's so scary about the bathroom? It's time you grow up. Look what you're doing to your mother!" Things would escalate into a yelling match from there, Eduardo countering with hostilities of his own. But nothing would change in the end, except that the atmosphere at home seemed to get worse and worse by the day.

Nicholas and Linda rarely argued, and they almost never had open disagreements over Linda's OCD symptoms and the impact her extreme avoidance had on their lives. But at times Nicholas still felt frustrated inside. For one thing, he was bothered that the two of them couldn't have a normal relationship with their granddaughter. He also didn't like Linda's rules about what movies and TV shows they could watch together and what photos could be displayed in their home. And he was very uncomfortable having to make up excuses to "cover" for Linda when she was feeling anxious. A part of Nicholas wanted to tell Linda how he felt. Maybe they could work things out and solve the problem together. But at the same time, he was afraid he wouldn't be able to find the right words. What if Linda mistook his frustration as a personal attack? OCD made her stressed out enough as it was; he didn't want to risk making things worse. So he figured it would be best to just go along with things despite feeling dissatisfied.

Although Ben often gave in to Ariel and helped with checking and providing reassurance, he, like Nicholas, was frustrated. Yet Ben often dealt with his frustrations by being sarcastic with Ariel and taking little jabs at her here and there. If Ariel became upset, he would tell her that he loved her and was just making "harmless jokes." Ben would also go behind Ariel's back and bad-mouth her to his friends. It seemed easier to laughingly mock her problems with OCD in front of his buddies than to directly confront Ariel about them. When this finally got back to Ariel, she was very hurt. Although he told Ariel that he was just "blowing off steam," Ben felt very guilty.

How do you relate with your relative when OCD symptoms rear their ugly head? What do you say and how do you say it? The box below describes four styles of communication: passive, aggressive, passive–aggressive, and assertive. Because of the nature of OCD, and how it affects family dynamics, I'd be willing to bet that you often use the first three styles, perhaps switching between them in different situations. But these styles aren't beneficial and can even worsen relationship stress and conflict. That's why, in this chapter, I'll help you use the most supportive communication style: assertiveness. And I'll refer back often to the assertiveness strategies provided here throughout the rest of this book. Assertiveness will help you successfully set boundaries, resolve conflicts and power struggles, and provide support as you take steps to alleviate the effects of OCD on your family.

The Four Communication Styles

Passive—Giving in to others no matter how much it inconveniences you and putting your own feelings and wishes aside so you can avoid conflict and keep everyone happy.

Aggressive—Intimidating or invalidating others, without thinking about their feelings and wishes, so you get what you want.

Passive–aggressive—Expressing feelings of resentment and trying to get what you want, but in a subtle, indirect, or backhanded way so you're not really owning your feelings.

Assertive—Showing respect for others while also standing up for yourself by listening thoughtfully, politely letting others know your feelings and wishes, and tactfully taking a stand when you disagree.

What Is Assertive Communication?

Assertiveness is the most supportive way to communicate with your loved one because it involves expressing that you genuinely understand his distress, but also that you intend to guide him toward better managing OCD-related anxiety. You make it clear that you are confident in his ability to manage distress without going on the attack or demanding that he change his behavior. This reduces conflict (in the long-run), validates your loved one's struggles, and improves his (and your own) self-esteem. Communicating assertively has many benefits, including cultivating mutual respect between you and your relative, feeling good about yourself and your relative, and reducing accommodation and other unhealthy family patterns that play into OCD. Assertiveness is many sided, which is why I've dedicated an entire chapter to teaching you the various aspects of this communication style. The first step is getting into the assertive mindset.

Getting into the Assertive Mindset

Communicating assertively with your loved one won't always be easy, but having the right mindset will make things go more smoothly. Fear often keeps people from acting assertively. Maybe you act passively because you're afraid of pushing your relative to face her fears. Or maybe you're worried she'll retaliate with anger and hostility if you stand up to her. At the root of these fears is a set of passive attitudes and beliefs that you'll want to throw out, such as the following:

- "It's awful when my loved one is upset with me."

- "My loved one's needs are more important than my own."

- "My loved one is fragile and can't handle too much anxiety, uncertainty, or conflict."

- "It's my job to make sure my family member with OCD never experiences any anxiety, distress, or other difficulties in life."

- "It's better to just 'go with the flow' and keep the peace, rather than confronting my loved one about OCD."

- "I'm not good at confrontations."

At the other end of the spectrum are thinking patterns that may lead you to be aggressive and demanding toward your relative. Perhaps you don't fully realize the challenges she faces or even believe OCD is a legitimate problem to begin with. Maybe it seems that using your power is the only way to get her to change. Do you find yourself agreeing with any of these statements?

- "Yelling is the only way to get my wife to act normally."
- "OCD is just a way for my partner to get attention."
- "She can (and should) just 'get over it.'"
- "My kid is a wimp—he shouldn't be so afraid."

To have success with assertiveness requires a mindset of its own. You'll need to realize that, like everyone else, you have a right to your own feelings, beliefs, and opinions—and the right to express them. This includes your right to say no. You also have the right to ask for what you want. And it's OK not to have your loved one's approval all the time. In fact, she's likely to disapprove of some of your new ways of helping her manage OCD—and she has every right to. When your family member becomes angry, remember this is driven by her obsessional fear. So rather than taking it personally or worrying that you'll cause an irreparable rift in your relationship, try to see it as an opportunity for her to get better at coping with anger and anxiety. In the end, you'll all be much happier when she learns how to better manage OCD.

On the flip side, assertiveness means keeping in mind that although you can *ask* for what you want, you won't always *get* it—and shouldn't expect to. After all, you can't control your loved one's behavior: what he says, how he acts, or what he thinks. Assertiveness, therefore, means recognizing that your loved one (no matter how old) gets to make decisions for herself, even if she sometimes disobeys your wishes, makes bad decisions, and has to face difficult consequences. You'll find it easier to be assertive when you stop trying to control your loved one and think in terms of *preferences* ("Things would be *better* if she decided to get treatment") instead of *demands* ("She *must* do the right thing and get treatment").

Finally, it's important to acknowledge the facts about anxiety, unwanted thoughts, and uncertainty that you've learned in Chapter 6. To successfully assert yourself with your loved one you'll need to remember that anxiety and fear are unpleasant but not harmful, obsessional thoughts are completely safe even if the ideas in them are disagreeable, and uncertainty is a normal part of life that every human being deals with. In short, it will be important that you view your family member with OCD as durable and resilient, rather than feeble or fragile.

How to Communicate Assertively

I *Statements*

"*I* statements" are the building blocks of assertive communication. They help you speak up for yourself in an honest and respectful way. When you start a sentence with "I . . . ," you're in the best position to let your relative know if you're upset about something without making accusations or putting her down. You're also in a good position to communicate your confidence in her ability to manage anxiety, obsessions, and uncertainty even though it might be difficult. Let's look at some examples of *I* statements and see how to construct them, and then you'll learn how to apply them in communicating with your loved one.

The box on the following page shows some sample *I* statements for different situations involving family members with OCD. As additional examples, Eduardo's father could have told Eduardo, "I realize you're afraid of contamination, but I'm also troubled that your mother has to clean your room and bathroom every morning." Nicholas might have said something like the following to Linda: "It's not easy for me to say this because I love you and don't want to upset you, but I don't like having to follow these OCD rules. I want us to have a closer relationship with our granddaughter, and I know you're capable of it. I would like for us to make some changes." Finally, rather than talk behind her back, Ben might say the following to Ariel: "I'm frustrated about these nightly checking rituals. And I don't like having to leave work in the middle of the day to provide reassurance because of OCD. I would like us to find a way to keep this from interfering with our marriage."

There's no one best *I* statement for a particular situation. In fact, you might be able to think of different (or better) ones for the scenarios in the box on the next page. What *is* important, though, is that your *I* statements stick to these guidelines:

- Acknowledge only the *facts* of the situation—what you can perceive with your five senses. This does not include your *interpretation* of your child's motives or your *opinion* of your partner's intentions.

- Acknowledge that how *you* feel about the situation is your own point of view and not necessarily how your loved one sees it.

Sample I *Statements*

Situation	I statement
Your child with OCD asks you the same questions over and over for reassurance.	"I've already answered that question, and it's not helpful for me to answer it again. It sounds like you're having a hard time with the uncertainty. Is there another way I can help you get through this?"
Your partner/spouse becomes upset because you did not follow her rules about avoiding contamination.	"I understand you're upset that I didn't take off my shoes before coming into the house this time; but I'm no longer going to follow OCD's rules. I realize this might make you afraid of contamination, but I also know how strong you are, and I'm confident you can manage this."
You're angry with your child because he's making everyone late for school by getting stuck with checking rituals.	"I realize you're worried about making sure the lights are off, but I'm also upset that we're late for school again and that the rituals are affecting your brother and sister, too. I hope we can work together to make changes so this doesn't happen again."
Your adult daughter asks that you remove all religious symbols from inside the home because they trigger her blasphemous obsessions.	"I know it's upsetting to you when you see a religious symbol and it provokes unwanted thoughts about God. It must be very frightening, and I hate that it's such a problem for you. But these symbols also mean a lot to me and the rest of the family, and I don't want to hide them. I also know you're strong and that you'll get through the distress. I'm here if you'd like my encouragement."
Your relative successfully resisted a compulsive urge in a situation that usually triggers compulsions.	"I'm very proud that you didn't wash your hands after throwing away that piece of trash. I know how difficult that must have been, and I'm very happy to see you succeed. You see, you can do this!"

- State your viewpoint in a way that doesn't blame or put down your family member—even if he really *is* to blame. It might be tempting to finger-point, but this will only put him on the defensive and make him not want to cooperate with you. A good rule of thumb is to try avoiding the word *you*.

- Let your loved one know you have confidence in her ability to manage anxiety, intrusive thoughts, and uncertainty.

Using the DEAR Method

Now, think about the various situations in your family or relationship where using a more assertive style could be helpful. Suppose you want to inform your son that you've decided not to buy special soap for his showers anymore. Maybe you want to say no when your wife asks you to help with rituals or provide reassurance. Perhaps you need to tell your daughter that you no longer want to help with her avoidance of objects that remind her of violence. The acronym DEAR provides a helpful way to structure assertive communication and incorporate *I* statements:

D *Define* **the problem.** Begin by explaining the issue to your loved one, but make sure you stick to objective facts. Simply state what you perceive as the problem. For example, Nicholas might say, "Linda, we have not been able to spend time together with our beautiful granddaughter. The rest of the family is wondering what's wrong, and I've had to make up excuses to help keep the OCD thoughts a secret."

E *Express* **your feelings.** Next, use *I* statements to let your relative know how you feel without finger-pointing or directly assigning blame. Try to word this so that your family member can relate to what you're going through. For example, "I don't like this situation at all. It really hurts me to lie to our kids about it." Make sure you don't substitute an *opinion* for a *feeling* ("I feel that you're just being irrational"). In other words, don't use *you* statements disguised as *I* statements. You'll only put your relative on the defensive and lose any chance of cooperation.

A *Ask* **for what you want.** Don't expect your relative to read your mind. So, in a fair, concise, and firm way, tell her your wish. But rather than assuming that you can control her behavior, state this as a *preference*, not a *command*. Also, express that you understand how having OCD makes your request seem frightening. For example, "I realize it might be frightening, but I would like to invite everyone, including Emma, to our house for dinner this week."

R **Provide** *reinforcement*. This means letting your loved one know that you appreciate her help and that you're confident she'll be able to manage the situation even if she feels anxious. A good way to do this is to describe the positive consequences of cooperating with your wish. For example, "I appreciate your cooperation even though it means you will probably feel uncomfortable. I love you, and I know you're strong. I know you'll get through this, and I will do everything I can to support you so that being with the baby gets easier."

Resolving Standoffs and Avoiding Conflicts

You can't control your loved one's behavior, and even being assertive doesn't guarantee he'll change his mind and do what you want him to. In most cases, OCD-related fear plays a big role in whether or not he cooperates. The *passive* response here is to give up, give in, and accommodate this fear. On the other hand, the *aggressive* response would be anger. But these approaches only make things worse in the long run. Instead, here are some assertive strategies you can use to tactfully resolve standoffs and avoid conflicts. They'll also help you sidestep being drawn into more accommodation. Of course, even using these tactics doesn't guarantee you'll get cooperation. But at least you'll know you've stuck up for yourself, tried your best, and probably garnered some respect from your loved one for doing so (even if he doesn't show it).

Broken record technique. This strategy involves calmly but firmly restating your point each time your family member tries to derail your assertiveness. For example, if your son protests, argues, or tries to change the subject, politely acknowledge that you've heard what he said, but stay on message and don't argue back or get diverted. Instead, become a "broken record" by using the same words over and over in slightly different sentences. You'll probably feel most comfortable using this technique when there is an implicit power differential, such as with your child. If you're using it with a partner or spouse, be sure to be courteous and respectful of the equality in your relationship. Here's an example in which a parent is using this technique with her daughter, who is afraid of contamination from her younger brother's clothes:

DAUGHTER: I saw *my* clothes in the same pile as Evan's. Did you wash them together!? You know mine can't touch his!

PARENT: Sweetie, because I want to help you get better, I've decided to stop washing your clothes separately from your brother's. It also takes me twice as long and wastes water when I wash them separately. I know this will upset you because you're afraid of contamination, but I want to help you learn that you're strong and don't need to avoid your brother's things just because OCD tells you so.

DAUGHTER: No! You can't do that to me!

PARENT: I love you and I want to help you learn that you don't have to listen to OCD's rules. *I'm* not going to listen to them anymore either.

DAUGHTER: But Evan picks his nose and rubs his hands on his clothes! Do you want me to get sick?

PARENT: (*Not getting drawn into a debate about whether she'll actually get sick*) I understand that you're anxious about this, but I love you and I want to help you see that you don't have to listen to OCD's rules. I've decided to stop too.

DAUGHTER: You're a horrible parent! If you *really* loved me, you'd wash our clothes separately and make me feel better.

PARENT: (*Calmly, and without responding to the personal attack*) I understand you're anxious. By not washing your clothes separately I'm helping you realize that you can get through the anxiety on your own. I'm not listening to OCD's rules anymore.

Turning the tables. When a standstill is reached in your conversation, one assertive move is to point this out and ask your loved one how *she* thinks the problem should be resolved. The parent in the example above, for instance, might say, "It looks like we're going around in circles here. I know you're upset and feeling anxious, but playing into OCD's rules for avoidance is not the answer for helping you. Plus, it takes up my time and ends up wasting water and detergent. Those things cost money. So, how do *you* think we should handle this?" When you try turning the tables, you might just get a compromise you can live with. But be prepared to continue your assertive role (perhaps using the *broken record technique*) if your family member suggests something you don't wish to go along with.

Time-outs. If you sense your loved one becoming angry, an assertive move is to refuse to continue the discussion. Instead, suggest a "time-out" to calm down. You might say, "I can see you're very upset right now. Let's continue this discussion later." Use the same strategy if you feel *yourself* becoming angry. You don't want to become overly emotional, because it's harder for you to think clearly and maintain your assertive stance. Try saying something like "I understand what you're saying, but I need some time to think it over" or "I'm not ready to talk about this right now. Let me find you in a little while."

Pointing out the process or the emotion. As alluded to earlier, your relative might respond to your assertiveness by trying to change the subject, threatening you, or drawing you into a debate or power struggle. For example, the girl with obsessional fears of her brother's clothes began dredging up disagreements from the past and calling her mother nasty names. If this occurs, the best course of action is to calmly point out what's happening in the conversation (that is, the *process*) and bring it back to what you wanted to discuss. For instance, you could say, "We're getting off the topic. We were talking about how to handle the situation with the laundry" or "I know you're upset about these past issues, and we can talk about them another time. Right now, we're discussing the laundry issue" or even "That sounds like a threat. I understand you're feeling angry, but it's a problem for me to do your laundry separately from your brother's." Importantly, don't let yourself get pulled into arguments over who is right and who is wrong.

If your loved one becomes quiet or teary-eyed, point this out as well: "I can see this is hard for you to talk about. I wonder what's making you feel uncomfortable." This strategy also works if the other person responds to your assertiveness by trying to make a joke ("Jokes are getting us off the topic— we're talking about the laundry right now") or by splitting hairs with you about whether your concerns are legitimate ("That's not the point. We've gotten off the topic"). If your loved one responds to your new way of dealing with OCD by becoming angry or spouting insults ("You're a terrible parent" or the like), don't take it personally. It usually means she knows that she's been outmatched and doesn't have much of an argument left.

Assertive Body Language

Believe it or not, your body language—the unspoken (nonverbal) communication we all use in everyday face-to-face encounters—can be *more* powerful than what you say out loud. That's why using assertive body language is so important. Just like your words, body language influences how people respond to you. It can make the difference between getting what you want and being taken advantage of. Here are some tips and suggestions for using assertive body language.

Eye contact. Make this a priority—it's probably the most important nonverbal way to communicate. Looking your loved one in the eye shows you're confident and respectful. But remember, it's not a staring contest! Don't glare—this will make her uncomfortable. Remain relaxed and occasionally look away. Also keep in mind that looking down too much suggests you're not sure of yourself. It sends the signal that you can be taken advantage of.

Posture, distance, and angling. Stand up straight when you need to be assertive. You'll feel more confident than if you're slouching forward. This tells your loved one, "What I'm saying is important." Angle yourself toward the person as well. She'll take this as a sign that you want to engage and have a dialogue. If you're angled away, she's sure to think you distrust her. Finally, don't fold your arms across your chest; it gives the signal that you're not open to communicating. Use arm and hand gestures to emphasize the importance of your feelings and wishes. But don't talk too much with your hands; it's a sign of nervousness. And too much (and very strong) hand gesturing can be a sign of aggression.

Facial expressions. Make sure your expression is consistent with what you're saying and how you're feeling. If you're giving a compliment, smile. If you're upset, don't. Your face should be sending the same message as your words.

Your tone of voice. Although it's not exactly a part of body language, your tone influences how your relative will receive what you're saying. When you speak in a deliberate way using a quiet tone and lower (deeper) pitch, you come across as more in control and self-confident, and your words are taken more seriously than if you speak in a higher, louder voice, which suggests that you're unsure of yourself.

Listening Assertively

Let's say your son has an obsessional fear of the number 13 and you're explaining to him that you'll no longer be helping him avoid that number. But then he suddenly blows up and accuses you of not understanding and never listening to a word he says. He stomps off angrily to his room, and your attempt to be assertive fails. But you know the number 13 isn't really dangerous—it's just a silly superstition, right? How could your son be so irrational?

An important part of being supportive is accepting that OCD makes your relative feel as if there's a dire threat that needs to be dealt with, even if *you* disagree that such a threat really exists. What's more, because the fight-or-flight response prioritizes threats over most anything else, his fear will seem more important to him than what you're trying to say. That's why it pays to practice *assertive listening,* which means trying to see things from his perspective (again, this is not the same thing as *agreement*). In the end, this can boost cooperation because your relative will be more willing to work with you when he feels you've heard him out and understand what he's going through. Listening is a lot more powerful than most of us believe. And more complicated. Here's how you can listen more assertively to your family member.

Focus. It seems obvious, but when you're dealing with OCD your mind might be going a million miles an hour in all different directions. Rest assured, though, your relative will sense it if your attention drifts away. So stay focused and show that you're interested in listening—even if you think you know what he's going to say (*and even if you disagree*). This will help you hear better and let him see that you're tuned in. Use the assertive body language I just described and be sure not to scowl, sigh, or look around the room or out the window. Clearly, this is also not the time to check your watch, phone, or e-mail. If the surroundings are distracting, you might even offer to continue the conversation in a quieter place.

Don't interrupt. Sure, it's hard to listen when your relative is saying things you disagree with. And it's difficult to resist stepping in with logic and trying to solve her problems. On the other hand, she's unlikely to listen to you in the way you want until she feels that you understand her. This means one of you has to be the one to demonstrate your understanding first. Since you can't control your loved one's behavior, the assertive and supportive move is for you to be the one to listen first.

Don't judge or challenge. Avoid disputing or invalidating your family member's views and feelings. For example, don't say things like "That's ridiculous!" or "There's no reason to be so afraid." In addition, "why" questions are likely to put your loved one on the defensive because she'll feel like she has to justify her position. Whether you agree or not, try to accept that *she's* got reasons for feeling afraid.

Be patient and don't practice a rebuttal. Your loved one won't feel like he's been listened to if it's clear you're impatiently awaiting your turn to speak.

So try not to let your body language reflect your eagerness. In addition, try not to think too much about your comeback while your relative is still speaking. If you're mentally preparing or rehearsing your response, you're not listening to what he's saying. A good strategy is to pretend there will be a test on what your relative is telling you!

Understand the take-home messages. As you're listening, try to take note of the main ideas your family member wants to get across to you. If you're not sure you understand what she's saying, it's OK to ask for clarification (for example, "I'm not sure what you mean. Can you help me understand that?").

When Your Loved One Has Finished Speaking

Once your loved one has finished speaking, the assertive response is to show that you've been listening by acknowledging his perspective, opinions, and emotions. One simple way to demonstrate this is by restating what he said. Eduardo's father, for example, might respond as follows: "Eduardo, I heard you say you're very afraid that harmful germs from outside the house have been spread onto our furniture. And you're afraid to come out of your room because you don't want to have to go through your showering ritual if you feel contaminated. So it's easier for you to stay in your room."

A slightly more complex response is to *paraphrase* what your relative says, restating the message using slightly different words. For example, you might say, "It sounds like you're scared that our furniture has germs from somewhere else that might be dangerous. And staying in your room is the only way to make sure you don't get those germs on you; because if you even thought that you did, you'd have to take a long shower to feel better." The idea here is to demonstrate that you have not only heard what your relative said but understood him well enough to be able to express the same thought using your own words. This is *not* the time to jump in and make suggestions. All you need to do is acknowledge that you've received the message your loved one is sending.

Catch Your Relative Doing Something Right!

Whenever possible, be aware of your loved doing something positive and then praise her for it. Letting her know how you feel by giving compliments will make her feel good, which in turn raises everyone's spirits. *I* statements can be helpful here, too. Rather than saying, "*You* did a great job getting ready for school on time," say something like "I was really happy with how you got yourself ready for school on time this morning, especially how you didn't need any help with getting dressed." And make sure to direct your praise toward what your relative *did* ("Xavier, you did a great job with not asking for reassurance all day!"), not at who he *is* ("Xavier, you're a really great guy!"). Your loved one is much too complex to be described by a single adjective.

At the same time, be careful not to overdo the compliments. If you're always dishing out large portions of praise, it will mean less and less to your loved one and she may even grow tired of hearing it. Also, make sure your compliments fit the achievement. That is, make sure the amount of praise you give, and how you give it, is appropriate. Some achievements (such as trying out a difficult exposure task or going an entire day without any rituals) are worth getting very excited about, while others (such as reducing shower time from 1 hour to 50 minutes) deserve a more measured response.

Practice, Practice, Practice!

Assertiveness is a skill, and like any other skill, it requires work and practice. I encourage you to keep a lookout for when others act assertively. Make a mental note of how they approach situations, what they say, and how they say it. You might interview them to find out. And it's OK to use a gradual approach. First, try being more assertive in easy situations. Then, when you're feeling more comfortable, challenge yourself to try it under more and more difficult circumstances with your family member with OCD. But whatever the outcome, don't beat yourself up. When you're unsuccessful—and this happens to just about everyone at some point—use it as a learning experience. Analyze the situation and ask yourself what you might do differently next time. With practice, you'll be able to use assertiveness to your advantage, including when working through the remainder of this book.

You've now got the foundation of knowledge and communication skills that you'll need to start reducing accommodation in order to support your relative with OCD and improve the overall atmosphere in your home. In Part III, I'll help you do this step by step. You'll get plenty of tactical advice and suggestions, and read lots of examples and illustrations, to help you get the best possible results from your efforts!

PART III

Reducing
OCD's Influence
Step by Step

8

Taking Stock of Your Situation

Now that you've got a clear understanding of how OCD works, how it gets entangled in relationships, and how it's treated, it's time to put all of this information to work and begin taking steps to turn things around in your household. The chapters in Part III are devoted to helping you get out from under OCD and promote a happier, healthier home environment even if your relative isn't ready to try treatment. But the changes you'll be making will also help your loved one develop more self-confidence and better manage obsessional fears and compulsive urges. More confidence and less fear in turn will reduce the negative impact OCD has on you, your family, and your relationships. Perhaps your loved one will decide to embrace these long-term benefits and cooperate with your agenda. Who knows? It might just give him the push he needs to decide that seeking professional help is worthwhile. If he is seeing a therapist, you can use this information to help you support his treatment.

You know that the anxiety, obsessions, and uncertainty involved in OCD are not harmful, and in fact are normal and commonplace, but I'm not saying the process of addressing them with your relative is easy. Some of my suggestions in the next several chapters might seem uncomfortable, "drastic," or even "radical" to you. So keep your mind open and remember that you're reading this book because what you've tried before hasn't been successful. It's time for a new approach to managing the situation with OCD in your home. The silver lining to all of this is that it often doesn't take very long to begin seeing real results, so I recommend making this process a priority for the next few months.

Your first step is to take stock of the situation and figure out exactly what needs to change. The legendary author and motivational speaker "Zig" Ziglar once said, "If you aim at nothing, you'll hit it every time." With this in mind, we'll begin by assessing the situation and identifying the patterns of accommodation that are occurring in your home so that you know where to take aim.

How Does OCD Impact Your Household?

In Part I of this book you read about the many ways OCD affects not only your loved one who has the disorder but also you and other people in your family. By exploiting your natural tendency to care for your loved ones, OCD draws close relatives and significant others into its web of obsessions, compulsions, and avoidance. Sure, you're protecting your relative from anxiety and the frustration or embarrassment of rituals, but then these become *your* problems. What's more, if you're always providing this protection, your loved one never gets the chance to learn that she can manage better than both of you think she can. So the vicious cycle goes on and on and leads to frustration, disruptions in day-to-day life, more OCD symptoms, and so on.

Finding your way out of this web begins with analyzing the situation. Start by looking at the big picture and completing the Impact of OCD Rating Form on pages 103–104 (you can also download this and the other forms in this chapter; see the information at the end of the Contents). The questions on this form will help you reflect on the degree to which your relative's OCD symptoms are currently affecting your family or relationship. Simply mark the appropriate box to indicate the extent to which your loved one's obsessions and compulsions lead to problems in these different areas of life. Depending on whether it's your partner, an adult son or daughter, or a child with OCD, some of these questions will apply more than others—and that's OK. This information will help you make important decisions about what to target to improve the quality of life in your household. And as you progress, you'll want to come back to this form (perhaps every month or two) to see how much of a difference your hard work is making.

Note that if your relative is working with a therapist, one part of the assessment process will be to identify the ways you and other household members have been accommodating OCD. So you may already have such a list compiled with the therapist, or you might show the therapist this chapter to see whether it makes sense to integrate the forms I provide into the therapy and homework.

Impact of OCD Rating Form

How much does your loved one's OCD lead to the following?

Type of problem	Not at all	A little	Somewhat	A lot	Extremely
Relational problems					
Arguments with your child	☐	☐	☐	☐	☐
Arguments with spouse/partner	☐	☐	☐	☐	☐
Arguments among siblings	☐	☐	☐	☐	☐
Reduced attention to others at home due to focus on OCD	☐	☐	☐	☐	☐
Reduced positive experiences with your loved one	☐	☐	☐	☐	☐
Problems with work or school					
Lateness	☐	☐	☐	☐	☐
Poor grades	☐	☐	☐	☐	☐
Problems performing at work	☐	☐	☐	☐	☐
Unemployment or job loss	☐	☐	☐	☐	☐
Problems with social or leisure time					
Avoidance of certain places	☐	☐	☐	☐	☐
Reduced interactions with others	☐	☐	☐	☐	☐

(continued)

Type of problem	Not at all	A little	Somewhat	A lot	Extremely
Problems with social or leisure time (continued)					
Time wasted on OCD	☐	☐	☐	☐	☐
Disruption of activities	☐	☐	☐	☐	☐
Trouble planning activities	☐	☐	☐	☐	☐
Reduced interest in social activities	☐	☐	☐	☐	☐
Problems around the house					
Chores don't get done	☐	☐	☐	☐	☐
Routines are disrupted	☐	☐	☐	☐	☐
There's lots of wasted time	☐	☐	☐	☐	☐
Problems with personal self-care					
Personal hygiene is neglected	☐	☐	☐	☐	☐
You feel tired/ fatigued	☐	☐	☐	☐	☐
Problems with sleeping	☐	☐	☐	☐	☐

Impact of OCD Rating Form *(continued)*

Analyzing Accommodation

Next, it's time to zero in and gather more in-depth and specific information so you can decide on personally tailored goals for effectively supporting your loved one. Think about it: if your clothes don't fit right, you take them to a tailor. But the tailor needs to measure you before making any alterations. Just like our bodies, OCD symptom accommodation takes different forms. And pinpointing the various ways you (and others) respond to your loved one's OCD symptoms is the key to designing a support program that fits your particular needs. This self-analysis will require a lot of thought, so I recommend going slowly and carefully. Also, you'll get the most benefit if you use a pencil or pen and write your answers down, rather than just "doing it in your head." There's something about writing that forces you to think more clearly and carefully about your answers. And although you're probably already aware of the main accommodation behaviors, in working through this exercise you might identify other behaviors and patterns that you didn't recognize.

Identifying Accommodation Patterns in Your Home

This chapter includes the forms needed to complete a full analysis of accommodation behaviors. Start with the Identifying Accommodation Worksheet on the next page, which is designed to help you recognize various forms of accommodation that you (and perhaps others in your home) might be engaging in because of your loved one's OCD symptoms. As you read the descriptions of each form of accommodation below, write your own examples in the appropriate spaces on the worksheet.

Providing help with rituals. List ways that you (or others) directly or indirectly help your relative carry out compulsive rituals. Ben, for example, checked that the doors were locked to reduce Ariel's obsessional fear of burglaries. Sometimes they checked together, and other times he'd initiate the checking on his own. Eduardo's mother engaged in cleaning rituals for Eduardo. The box on page 107 includes additional examples of accommodation for different types of rituals.

Giving reassurance. Reassurance seeking is a particular type of ritual, but one that often draws accommodation from family members so it's worth paying special attention to. In what ways do you reassure your loved one to calm his obsessional fear and uncertainty? Xavier's father repeatedly answered Xavier's questions about sin and punishment from God. Nicholas

Identifying Accommodation Worksheet

1. Providing help with rituals:

2. Giving reassurance:

3. Helping with avoidance:

4. Assisting with minor tasks and decisions:

5. Taking on responsibilities:

6. Allowing or helping with unacceptable or extreme behavior:

Common Ways That Family Members Accommodate OCD Rituals

Type of ritual	Accommodation patterns
Washing/cleaning	• Washing, showering, or cleaning for a loved one • Changing clothes after visiting "contaminated" places • Doing extra loads of laundry • Preparing food in an atypical way • Providing cleaning supplies (or money to buy them) • Allowing time for rituals • Making excuses for lateness because of rituals • Cleaning or wiping down items brought into the home
Checking	• Performing checks for a loved one • Checking together • Excessive proofreading • Providing excuses to others for lateness because of excessive checking rituals
Ordering	• Helping with putting things in their "proper" or "perfect" order, place, or arrangement • Helping to "balance" something out
Reassurance seeking	• Providing reassurance by answering frequent questions about safety, risk, illness, probabilities, sexuality, bad luck, morality, religion, and the like • Helping with repeated Internet searches to find information about obsessional fears • Helping with efforts to seek reassurance from authority figures (such as repeatedly driving a loved one to see an expert) • Listening to compulsive apologizing, explaining, or confessing
Religious rituals	• Excessively repeating religious ceremonies together • Excessive praying with a spouse or child
Mental rituals	• Helping with thinking positive thoughts • Helping with trying to remember or review things

gave Linda frequent reassurance that she was neither a pedophile nor a danger to her grandchild. Here are some additional examples:

- Assuring your spouse that she'd have noticed if she hit a pedestrian with her car
- Reminding your daughter that she already checked the stove three times and it was off
- Reassuring your son that washing his penis is not the same as masturbation
- Assuring your adult child that she is not a violent person
- Explaining to a loved one with contamination fears that he's unlikely to get sick from touching _____
- Answering the same (or similar) questions over and over for your loved one

Helping with avoidance. Do you (or others in your home) assist your loved one with avoiding certain places, objects, numbers, colors, words, or people that provoke obsessional fear or compulsive rituals? Nicholas helped Linda avoid reminders of their granddaughter by refraining from using Emma's name and making up excuses to cover for Linda so she could keep up her avoidance. In the box on the facing page, I've included further examples of how family members might help with avoidance related to different types of obsessions.

Assisting with minor tasks and decisions. Are there routine, everyday things your loved one is capable of doing, and decisions she is capable of making, that you (or other family members) either do yourself or try to make easier for your loved one? Ben, for example, locked doors for Ariel because she would get stuck checking over and over to make sure they were really locked. Here are other examples of this kind of accommodation:

- Cutting food for your daughter who is afraid to use knives because of her obsessional thoughts of stabbing people
- Picking things up off the floor for your wife with fears of contamination from floors
- Waking up your partner or an adult child (as if you have to be the person's alarm clock)

Common Ways That Family Members Accommodate Avoidance

Type of obsessions	Accommodation patterns
Contamination	• Opening doors, flushing toilets, and touching other things for the person with OCD • Agreeing to handle feared items so the person with OCD doesn't have to • Agreeing not to bring certain items into the home • Removing "contaminated" work clothes before entering the home • Agreeing to stay away from places or items believed to be contaminated • Testing things for a loved one to make sure they're safe or clean
Fears of harm or mistakes	• Agreeing to be the last one to leave the house to help with avoidance of feeling accountable • Driving for a partner to prevent him from having obsessions about accidents or pedestrians • Taking over paying bills • Agreeing to take over all child care responsibilities for a new baby to help avoid thoughts of harming the child
Incompleteness	• Keeping things arranged or balanced a certain way to prevent "not just right" feelings
Sex or violence	• Taking an out-of-the-way route to avoid passing stimuli that prompt obsessions (such as cemeteries) • Holding back from discussing certain topics or using words or numbers that trigger obsessional thoughts • Asking not to have a loved one's "bad luck" room number at a hotel • Keeping items that trigger obsessions (such as knives, books, or pictures) out of sight • Handling knives for someone with obsessions about violence • Agreeing to avoid certain movies or shows as a family or as a couple

- Making simple decisions for your adult son, such as when to wake up, what to eat, and which clothes to wear. (A mother made decisions like these for her son, who was afraid God would punish him for being selfish and prideful if he made decisions "too quickly and carelessly"; but they were taking him hours to make on his own.)

Taking on responsibilities. Perhaps there are more significant chores, tasks, and other responsibilities that you'd otherwise expect your relative to complete, but because she has OCD you bend over backward or change the regular routine so you (or others) can do them for her. Eduardo's mother, for example, cleaned Eduardo's room, made his bed, and prepared his food even though Eduardo was 17 and perfectly capable of completing these tasks. Here are more examples:

- Doing homework for your child
- Doing household chores (like taking out the trash) that are assigned to a member of the family with OCD
- Micromanaging school issues for your teenager
- Taking over all cooking responsibilities because of your partner's obsessional fear
- Making social or work-related phone calls (or writing e-mails) on behalf of your adult daughter
- Changing or bathing the baby because your spouse has obsessions about sex or harm
- Chauffeuring or running errands for your partner who's able to drive himself but has fears of hitting pedestrians

Allowing or helping with unacceptable or extreme behavior. This form of accommodation involves putting up with (or perhaps *helping* with) your loved one's undesirable or unusual requests and behaviors because she has OCD. Eduardo's mother, for example, permitted (and in fact helped) Eduardo to stay home from school and remain in his room. Quitting her job, waiting on Eduardo hand and foot (for example, cleaning his bathroom every day), buying games so Eduardo could be entertained, and putting up with his other extreme demands and rude outbursts were all forms of OCD accommodation. Nicholas was also accommodating when he put up with Linda's wishes that certain TV shows not be watched, their granddaughter's name not be mentioned, and the like. He would never agree to avoid such things if Linda didn't have OCD. Some other examples include:

- Allowing your son to make the rest of the family late while he completes rituals
- Giving in to demands that you change clothes before entering the house, avoid using certain furniture, go in certain rooms, or take extra showers
- Agreeing to not allow "contaminated" guests in the home
- Putting up with extremely disrespectful or destructive behavior
- Putting up with poor hygiene or extreme messiness caused by OCD
- Waking up early or going to bed late because of your relative's OCD
- Sleeping with your child or sleeping apart from your spouse because of OCD
- Moving to a new home because something about the old home provokes a family member's obsessional fear
- Keeping your son on the company payroll even though he rarely shows up for work
- Paying for (or buying things for) an adult relative who refuses to look for employment
- Allowing an adult child to live in your home if she's capable of living on her own

Keep in mind that it's sometimes tricky distinguishing accommodation patterns from beneficial ways you'd help and support a loved one in need. Calling your son's school to let them know he'll be absent is fine if your son is asleep in bed with the flu. But it's accommodating OCD if you call to say he's feeling too anxious to attend. Similarly, dividing up child care duties for your newborn is part of having an equitable relationship unless task division is one-sided and aligns with your spouse's OCD-related avoidance. If you're stuck trying to figure out whether something you're doing is accommodation, ask yourself if you're doing it because your relative has OCD. If you wouldn't do this for someone without the disorder, it's probably accommodation. Similarly, if what you're doing (or putting up with) seems excessive, repetitive, or unnecessary, or pushes the limits of what seems appropriate, it's likely accommodation and you should write it down on the worksheet.

When, Where, and How Often?

After identifying the forms of accommodation that occur in your relationship or family, you're ready to complete the Daily Accommodation Log on pages 113–114. Note that the log is made up of three columns: Time Period, Accommodation Behavior, and Situation. I've divided the Time Period column into sections for morning, afternoon, evening, bedtime/overnight, weekend, and "other" because accommodation often follows patterns that sync with these periods. Weekend and vacation or holiday routines tend to be different, so I've made those separate categories. During each phase of the day, record any accommodation behaviors (from the Identifying Accommodation Worksheet) that occur in the middle column. Remember these are things you (or other family members) do that make it easier for your loved one with OCD or that reduce or protect her from anxiety in the moment. In the Situation column on the right, describe any events that led to the particular instance of accommodation. Be aware that some accommodation behaviors may not be triggered by an actual event per se, but rather in anticipation of a particular circumstance or just as part of what's become the daily routine.

An example from Eduardo's mother's log appears on page 115. Notice that you don't have to write a book for each entry—after all, this is only for your use!

Keep track of accommodation every day for at least a full week before moving on to the next chapter. You can start a new log sheet for each day. I know it seems tedious, and I'm sure you want to begin making changes right away, but it's actually very important to take your time here (feel free to *read* ahead while you're keeping the logs; just hold off on taking *action* for now).

Why track accommodation for a full week? For one thing, it will allow you to notice which accommodation patterns recur daily and which ones are more sporadic—and we'll be prioritizing these differently when it comes to setting goals. And while you might *think* you're already aware of all the accommodation taking place, many couples and families I work with are surprised to see how much they'd been overlooking. Second, it's a fact that simply self-monitoring helps people change their behavior. So knowing you're supposed to write down every time you provide accommodation might just be the thing to help you hold back. Finally, keeping this log is a good way to track how much these patterns change over time. You'll hopefully see differences when you compare this week's logs to one you complete a few months from now.

Daily Accommodation Log

Day and date: _____

Time period	Accommodation behavior	Situation
Morning • Getting up • Getting dressed • Breakfast • Going to school/ work • Chores		
Afternoon • During school/work • At home • Lunch • Homework • Extracurricular activities • Social activities		
Evening • Dinner • Social activities • Family/couple time • Chores		

(continued)

Time period	Accommodation behavior	Situation
Bedtime/Overnight • Washing up/ showering • Going to bed • Sleeping • Sex/intimacy		
Weekend • Errands • Religious services • Social activities • Around the house • Family/couple activities		
Other • Travel/vacation • Holidays		

Sample Daily Accommodation Log
from Eduardo's Mother

Time period	Accommodation behavior	Situation
Morning • Getting up • Getting dressed • Breakfast • Going to school/ work • Chores	Got up at 5:30 A.M. to clean the bathroom for Eduardo Woke Eduardo up at 8 A.M. Fixed his breakfast and brought it to his room Cleaned his room while he was in the shower	Part of the regular morning routine
Afternoon • During school/work • At home • Lunch • Homework • Extracurricular activities • Social activities	Put up with name-calling and threats when I tried to tell Eduardo the lunch I made him wasn't contaminated Washed the refrigerator door for Eduardo Went out and bought Eduardo lunch from McDonald's	Eduardo knew his sister had touched the refrigerator without washing her hands and didn't want any food from the fridge today

Using the Information You've Gathered

After spending a week identifying and charting accommodation patterns, review the information you've gathered and pinpoint those situations and accommodation behaviors that get in the way, occur frequently, take up your time, create frustration, or prove costly. These are the patterns you'll need to address to help your family member become more independent, self-reliant, resilient, and self-confident. Keep the forms and logs you completed in this chapter handy, because we'll use them again in Chapter 11 to set specific goals for reducing accommodation.

The next step in the process, however, is to let your loved one know that you've decided to change how you respond to OCD. But speaking with your relative about how you plan to work toward ending the accommodation patterns you just identified can be a challenge. Perhaps, like many people I've worked with, you've hit roadblocks at this point in the past. He becomes very anxious and talks you out of making changes. She becomes angry and draws you into more accommodation. This is normal; and it's why I've included the next chapter, which will help you make sure your message (and your determination to follow through) gets through this time. I'll also arm you with strategies for dealing with negative reactions your family member might have when you deliver this message.

9

Preparing Your Loved One

Now that you've got a good sense of the patterns of accommodation that occur in your home and how detrimental they are, it's time to let your family member know that you're determined to end these routines, help him become more self-confident, and cultivate a healthier and more enjoyable atmosphere. In this chapter, I'll help you carefully develop and deliver this message in the form of an "announcement" or "declaration" to your loved one. Making your intentions known is just the first stage in the process of change. Once you've delivered your message, you'll work on setting boundaries and expectations with your loved one (Chapter 10) and then set more specific goals and develop a road map for reducing accommodation, which you'll follow step by step (Chapter 11).

For various reasons, many families and couples avoid talking about ending accommodation. To be successful, though, this time needs to be a true turning point. Let me therefore suggest reading through this entire chapter before you begin any conversations or announcements with your relative about the changes you're about to make. I'll help you get past the most common roadblocks to communicate successfully and effectively handle any pushback you encounter. I'll also help you get the support you might need, from your partner in communicating with a child and from someone outside the family if you need such support.

Making Sure Your Message Gets Through This Time

Why have things gone wrong when you've tried to talk to your relative about making changes in the past?

One possibility is that your timing's been off. Rather than waiting until things are relaxed in your home, perhaps you've confronted your family member in the heat of the moment. But if you're upset over another shouting match, missed event, or sleepless night dealing with OCD, you're likely to lose your cool or have trouble remembering what you really wanted to say. And your relative isn't ready to listen to you either—she's angry, anxious, or feeling bad about the situation.

Or maybe the problem's with the message itself. Are you too vague so that she doesn't know what to expect? Do you try to tell her what *she's* got to do differently rather than focusing on changing your own behavior? Is your message confrontational or critical as opposed to supportive and optimistic? Do you come across as unsure or unconvinced? Do you negotiate with your loved one? Do you lecture her or come across as angry? A "yes" answer to any of these questions might explain why past attempts to speak to your loved one about OCD haven't worked out well.

Whatever the reasons for difficulty in the past, what's going to be different this time is that your only mission is to communicate your message to your loved one. That's all. Don't worry about his reaction—or whether he even pays attention to you (he's probably paying careful attention even if it doesn't look that way). And discard any expectations that your declaration will instantly result in any changes. You're merely informing your loved one—in a clear, firm, and considerate way—that you plan to make some changes in how you handle OCD and accommodation. How he responds will be up to him (remember, you can't control his responses). So, here are some considerations as you begin to think about how you'll deliver your message:

What to Say

- Be genuine. Let your family member know that you love him and that you acknowledge his difficulty with OCD.

- Explain that you're making changes to your own behavior because as the parent/spouse/partner it's your job to help your loved one overcome problems.

- Be concrete about what you're planning to change. A hazy description will only add to your loved one's anxiety and uncertainty. I'll show you some examples later in this chapter.

- Keep the focus on what *you'll* be doing differently, not on what your relative needs to change. Never point the finger or tell him he's got to handle OCD better.

- Let your loved one know that you understand reducing accommodation will increase her anxiety but that she's strong and you're confident she'll be able to manage it.

- Say that you hope she'll work with you, even though you can't force her to cooperate.

- Let him know he can trust that you'll stick to your plan. If applicable, make it clear that both parents are on board or that you'll be recruiting help from people outside your family.

How to Say It

- Be concise and to the point rather than long-winded.

- It's OK to be firm and formal. This will help your relative see your declaration as a turning point and give it more weight and significance. It shows you're taking this seriously. Maintain a purposeful tone and don't become overly emotional.

- Even if you're frustrated, never appear as blaming, criticizing, or ridiculing. Rather, come across as genuinely concerned and determined to work hard to make everyone's life better in the end.

- Be confident. Know that your actions are loving and supportive—it's part of your responsibility as parent or partner, even if your relative objects or tries to make you think otherwise.

- Don't debate or negotiate. You've made up your mind about making changes, and you're determined to stick to your plan.

- Remember that you can control only your own behavior. Put yourself in this mindset: *I'm going to make changes that are meant to help you. I hope you'll cooperate, but I can't control how you respond.*

Tips for Success

- Timing is everything. Deliver your declaration when both you and your loved one are feeling relatively calm. Maybe she's in her room reading or watching a video. Maybe he's doing homework, listening to music, or just relaxing in front of the TV. This will help your relative focus on the message, rather than being distracted by anger or anxiety.

- Minimize other distractions. For example, don't do this while driving or try to squeeze it in during half-time of the game you're watching. Make sure other family members are occupied or looked after (or better yet, out of the house) so there are no interruptions.

- Create a written script of your declaration and have it with you. This will ensure you say everything you intended to say and avoid getting sidetracked if your relative tries to distract you. You can also give the written copy to your relative after you've made the declaration verbally.

- Rehearse your delivery of the message in front of a mirror or with someone else before approaching your relative with OCD.

- If you're a parent and you have a spouse or partner, deliver your message together. This will make it clear that you both agree with the plan and can't be split against each other (more on this later in the chapter).

- Sit down with your loved one in a nonconfrontational way, present your message, hand her the written copy, then give her a hug, tell her you're proud of her, and leave the room.

Sample Declarations

Here are five sample declarations you can use to construct your own message:

Eduardo's Parents' Declaration

"Eduardo, we love you very much and understand how afraid OCD makes you feel about bathroom germs and contamination. We know how it makes you afraid to come out of your room, interact with the rest of the family, and go to school. As your parents it's our responsibility to help you become independent, happy, and productive. And we're determined to do that for you. We admit that staying home with you, bringing food to your room, cleaning for you, and making sure everyone in the house follows OCD's rules hasn't worked. That's our fault, and so your father and I have decided to make changes in how we deal with OCD. In order to help you, we're going to stop giving in to the contamination fears. We will do this step by step, and we will talk with you about each new change when we're ready to make it. This will be challenging for you, but we also know you're strong enough to defeat OCD. We're not angry at you, and we're not trying to punish you. We just care too much to keep letting

OCD hurt you. We hope you'll work together with us, although we are prepared to move ahead with our plan either way."

Ben's Message to Ariel

"Ariel, I love you more than words can say. You and our family mean so much to me, and I know they mean everything you, too. I also know how much your obsessions make you anxious and that it seems like the only way out is to check over and over. But whenever you check—and whenever I check for you—there's never, *ever*, been any danger present. So, I now realize that when I "help" you with checking, it's really working against you. It makes you feel better for the time being, but the doubting gets worse in the long run. And as your husband, I can't ignore this anymore. So, I've decided that I'm going to work on providing the right kind of help from now on, which means helping you stand up to OCD, rather than doing rituals for you. I hope that we can work on this as a team—I know you're capable."

Xavier's Parents' Declaration

"Xavier, we hate seeing you suffer with the pain and uncertainty that your OCD causes you. Since you were young you have always come to us for advice and assurance, and as your parents we've always had the right words for you. But Mother and I also know that our behavior— answering your questions at all hours of the day or night, doing whatever we can to try to keep you feeling reassured, paying you even though you don't actually work at the store—only does you a disservice. You're an adult now, and it's our job to help you get better at managing OCD and back to being independent. That's why, after discussing it together, we've decided on some new policies in our house that will help you achieve these things. We will be changing the way we respond to the OCD symptoms so we can help you become self-sufficient. We have also decided not to keep this to ourselves anymore. We will be seeking out people in our community we think can help provide support. We'll let you know the details of these policies as we gradually put them in place, and although it might not be easy for you, we're very confident that you'll rise to the challenge and work with us. We love you very much."

Nicholas's Message to Linda

"Linda, you are the love of my life, and I am so proud that we are grandparents now! I also know how much your OCD thoughts upset you and make you think you've got to follow certain rules and avoid Emma. As much as I hate seeing you suffer with OCD, I'm not comfortable with how I've been handling things. I don't like lying to our family or putting up with OCD's rules. I realize it seems like the avoidance is necessary, but it's taking away from the joy of being grandparents, and I know *you* wish things were different too. So, I've decided I'm going to stop playing by OCD's rules—I hope *you'll* decide to do the same. I understand there will be times when you think about difficult things and become upset, and I'm sorry. But as your husband, I want to help you solve this problem the right way. You've always been strong—it's one of the things I love most about you. And I'm confident you have the strength to do this with me so that we can enjoy our wonderful family."

Brittany's Parents' Declaration

Brittany, an 11-year-old girl, has tapping compulsions that make her late for school and for appointments and that routinely hold up her family. Specifically, Brittany feels she has to tap all signs and notices posted on walls that she walks past. Her obsessional fear is that if she does not tap everything, she will cause bad luck for her family.

"Brittany, you are a smart, beautiful, and strong girl—and we love you very much. We know that OCD makes you think you've got to touch and tap every sign you walk past in order to prevent bad luck, and we realize it's a very difficult thing for you to ignore. But as your parents, it is our responsibility to help you solve problems. We know you've got what it takes to stand up to OCD, and we have decided we're going to help you do exactly that. From now on, we're going to do a better job of not letting OCD bully you or our family into missing out on important parts of life. We're not mad at you for having this problem, and we know that if you could choose to stop the rituals right now, you would. But now it's time for us to start helping you. We are sure that if we work together, we can beat this."

How Will Your Loved One Respond?
(And What You Should Do)

Your relative may welcome your message with interest and willingness. Maybe she'll be relieved and eager to cooperate because she's also been feeling like things need to change. When Nicholas informed Linda that he'd decided to stop accommodating her OCD, Linda understood. "You're right. I don't like how I've handled the OCD thoughts and avoidance, and I need to make changes too. I'm glad you're going to push me to do better," she told her husband. If this is your loved one's response, great! The following chapters will walk you through the next steps.

On the other hand, your family member might greet your announcement with hostility or other resistance. You're proposing to stop protecting him from fear and push him to do things he's been avoiding, so his opposition is understandable. He senses that life is about to get more difficult, and he's naturally apprehensive. Psychologists Eli Lebowitz and Haim Omer have identified the following reactions you're likely to encounter, along with excellent suggestions for how you can respond.

Begging and Bargaining

Xavier responded to his parents' announcement by trying to convince them that their plan would make things even worse. He also bargained with them: "I promise I'll start applying for jobs tomorrow. Please don't stop the reassurance. Just give me one more chance!" (something his parents had heard many times before). If your relative takes this route, understand that he's trying to deter you from following through with your plan. Your best option is to not engage in arguments or debates. Instead, use the assertiveness skills you learned in Chapter 7 to explain that you're not interested in discussing the matter any further at this time. If you fall into the trap of debating and trying to convince your relative that you are doing the right thing, you'll only send the message that you're not completely on board. And that will give him hope that you can be talked out of it. Xavier's mother, for example, calmly but clearly explained, "I've told you everything I have to say at this point. Your father and I will be thinking about what to do next, and we'll let you know when we have something more to tell you." Then she left the room.

Blame

Eduardo knew exactly how to turn the blame on his mother and make her feel guilty and upset: "You're a terrible parent! You're only doing this because you don't love me. You're making me hate you!" Because saying these things had worked in the past to get his mother to back off, it's no surprise that he used them again and again. But Eduardo's mother realized her son's harsh words were motivated by anxiety—not hate. So, as difficult as it was, she didn't let herself take them personally. She knew that what she was doing was for the best and so she didn't need to prove that she was a good parent or that she loved Eduardo. Being a confident, supportive, and loving parent sometimes means doing things that upset your child. In such instances, it's perfectly appropriate to let your loved one feel anxious and angry and say something like "I understand you don't like what I told you and I'm sorry you're angry, but this is very important to me."

Becoming Emotional

Ariel became emotional and began crying when Ben informed her of his plan to stop accommodating her OCD symptoms. Although crying can be a calculated strategy to guilt you into changing your behavior, it's usually a sign of true distress. Either way, it's important to resist any urge to give in or change your plan. Remember that your loved one's anxiety and distress are temporary and manageable, so think of this as an opportunity to help your relative learn that she can manage these emotions. Ben consoled Ariel with a hug and made sure to validate her feelings of anxiety, but also resisted the urge to change his plan.

Indifference and Inattention

Your loved one might respond as if she's unmoved or indifferent: "I don't really care what you do." She might avoid eye contact, pretend not to hear you, or hide out of sight. But rest assured she hears you loud and clear, so there's no need to repeat your message or demand that she listen more closely. In fact, if your relative begins to ignore you after you've approached her, try one time to get her attention back by politely saying, "There's something I'd like to talk to you about; could you please listen?" or "Please put down your phone; we need to speak with you." If the ignoring continues, proceed with saying what you planned to say without insisting that she pay attention. Don't try to take away any phones, computers, or other devices and never use physical force of any kind as this will only lead to angry or disruptive behavior. Remember that your job is merely to deliver your announcement—not force her to listen to you.

If your loved one leaves the room before you've finished, don't go after her. If she's within earshot, calmly continue with your message and then place the written copy someplace where she'll find it (such as on a bed or desk). If she's too far to hear you, simply leave the written declaration and walk away.

Verbal Threats

Although it's less common, your loved one may respond with threats of self-harm, suicide, and the like. Eduardo, for example, told his parents he would run away from home if they stopped accommodating his OCD. Such threats generally do not represent a serious risk. Most likely, they're a knee-jerk response to feeling anxious and the threat of losing control. Your loved one may also be testing you to see if you'll back down (as you might have done in the past). That said, these threats need to be handled carefully. In Chapter 12 you'll learn supportive ways to respond should your family member actually play this card.

Interruptions

Your child might heckle or mock you or make inappropriate gestures. But this, too, is driven by anxiety and fear rather than by disrespect. He's only trying to derail you and get you off message. So, as difficult as it seems, the best way to handle it is to ignore his antics and continue delivering your message calmly. If you lose your composure or demand that he stop, you'll only be playing into his hands and teaching him to use similar tactics whenever you try to address OCD in the future.

If your loved one destroys the written copy of your declaration (such as crumpling it into a ball and throwing it at you), ignore this too. She'll probably be intrigued enough to recover it and read it when you're not around. This reflects the ambivalence that I described in Chapter 5. Your loved one is fearful of change, but at the same time she's hopeful that things can get better.

Aggression

In rarer instances, your family member might act out and do any of the following:

- Scream at you to leave the room
- Curse at you
- Use other verbally abusive behavior
- Threaten to physically harm you
- Throw things at you
- Push or hit you

Here again, these actions are a reflection of anxious apprehension, and I recommend not responding to them at this point if at all possible (in Chapter 12, I'll provide suggestions for how to supportively manage severely aggressive behavior). Instead, calmly state your message, leave the written document, and leave the room without acknowledging the aggression. If you encounter more serious physical aggression that is impossible to ignore, calmly leave the written document and walk away from your relative without saying anything (then go read Chapter 12!). Remember that giving your family member the attention he's seeking will only reinforce the inappropriate behavior. Try to stay resolute and don't let your relative see how much it really bothers you (this might be a good time to take a break and do something for yourself or get some exercise to blow off some steam).

What's Next?

You've given your loved one the heads-up that changes are coming. Now it's time to use what you've learned so far in this book to begin supporting your family member with OCD by taking action and improving the daily conditions in your family or your relationship. In the next chapter, you'll learn how to set and maintain healthy boundaries and expectations. These are important because, as you'll see, they provide the structure you'll need for reducing accommodation. The process might be challenging at times, but in the end, with hard work and consistency, you'll reap long-term rewards for you, your relative, and your family.

Speaking of challenges, you'll find them easier to overcome the more support and collaboration you have from others. So before you communicate your plan to your loved one, carefully consider the information presented next.

Recruiting Support from Outside Your Family

Maybe you're the single parent of someone with OCD, and you're concerned about making changes without the help of another adult. Perhaps it's your spouse with obsessions and compulsions, and you feel you'll need support when it comes to reducing accommodation. Are there dependable people in your community but outside your nuclear family whom your loved one with OCD admires, respects, or seeks out for advice? Perhaps it's an aunt, uncle, or grandparent. Maybe there are close family friends who have known your loved one for a while, or perhaps clergy members, school guidance counselors, athletic coaches, or professionals such as doctors, dentists, or accountants. Lebowitz and Omer again suggest identifying one or more such individuals—we'll call them *advocates*—and enlisting their help to back you up through the process of changing how you respond to OCD.

Advocates can connect with your relative on a more formal level than you might be able to and keep lines of communication open when emotions run high. They can also help to manage crises or disruptive behavior as necessary and offer you moral support and encouragement when you're feeling challenged. Finally, advocates can provide your relative with rewards for progress by giving praise, tangible rewards, or just spending time together (as I'll describe in Chapter 10).

Addressing Concerns

If you're uncomfortable with the idea of involving someone from outside the family in your personal business, I understand. And you're not alone. Some of my own patients express the same feelings at first. Here are some common concerns and reservations.

What if my relative reacts negatively? Yes, your loved one might temporarily feel upset or embarrassed that the advocate knows about his disorder. But in the long run, when it's clear the advocate isn't there to be judgmental, and instead is dedicated to helping your relative (and the entire family) fare better, the relationship will be strengthened.

Isn't OCD our family's private business? Your family has a right to privacy—especially as it relates to sensitive issues such as mental health. At the same time, *you've* also got the right to pull out all the stops to support your relative and make your household a healthier place to live. The advocate is not there to shame your loved one, but rather to rally around him and help send the message that he is loved and cared for, that others believe in him, and that you're not going to give up on making things better.

Isn't this an admission of failure? The idea that you've failed as a parent or partner if you have to turn to members of your community for help and support is absolutely false. Not only that, it denies both you and your loved one helpful resources. It's a fact that many problems can't be solved within the limits of the immediate family—and there's no shame in turning elsewhere for help.

Choosing Your Advocates

Make a list of potential advocates—the more the better. Some of them will probably become more involved than others, and that's fine. And being an advocate requires no special training. You'll provide all the information they need (as I'll describe next). What's key is that they're willing to help support your loved one and are generally considerate, optimistic, warm, and thoughtful. They'll also need to be able to communicate firmly and assertively. When your relative sees others from outside the family conveying a message consistent with your own, it can have a strong impact. On the other hand, people who tend to be pessimistic, critical, and either overly lenient or overly pushy tend to make poor advocates.

When you're ready to contact potential advocates, be open and honest about your loved one's difficulties with OCD and how it's affecting your family or relationship. Let the advocate know that you're working to help your loved one overcome OCD and that it's recommended that you involve people outside your immediate family who may be willing to lend a hand. Clarify that if the person decides to help, you'll never ask him to sacrifice his own obligations or responsibilities. The first job of an advocate (once you make your declaration) is to connect with the person with OCD and let him know she's going to be involved. The advocate should convey that she is aware of OCD and how it affects the family, that your loved one is special to the advocate, and that she's interested in helping improve the situation, looks forward to this role, and will follow up in the future. This can be done in person, over the phone, through the mail, or by videoconferencing.

As an example, Xavier's parents enlisted Xavier's favorite pastor as an advocate. He stopped by Xavier's home on his way to work and told Xavier: "Xavier, your parents made me aware of the problems you're having with OCD and how they affect your whole family. You know that you're all very important to me. I care about you and your family a great deal. That's why I hate to hear that you're experiencing so much fear and suffering. Your mother and father asked me to lend a hand, and I want you to know that I'm here to give you support as you work through this with your family. I'm sure we'll be talking about this again sometime soon."

For Parents: Enhancing Teamwork

Having a son or daughter with OCD—whether a child or an adult—can strain a couple's relationship. But if you and your spouse or partner aren't working together as parents, that level of frustration and resentment increases exponentially. Do the two of you have different parenting styles? Do you disagree over how to respond when your child experiences obsessional fear or anxiety, or gets stuck doing compulsive rituals? Maybe one of you is more demanding and the other more permissive. I see such differences all the time in couples, but even so, it's critical that you present a unified front. With this in mind, here are some ways to optimize collaboration and teamwork.

Look for Common Ground

Even if one of you tends to be more lenient, the two of you want the same thing: for your loved one to become more confident and self-reliant. So, try to blend acceptance of your child's anxiety with confidence in her ability to manage it.

Be on the Same Team in Front of Your Child

Even if you disagree on how to handle OCD, you've got to be on the same team in front of your child. Develop some house rules that you can both agree on, such as no name-calling, cell phones off during meals, and no screen time until after homework is completed. Make sure to inform your spouse if an issue has come up around OCD. For example, "Honey, I wanted you to know that I told Peyton I would not wash her laundry again." And do this in front of your child to send the message that she can't play you off one another.

Discuss Your Differences and Make Decisions in Private

If you disagree with something your partner said or did, wait until your child isn't around to bring it up, using assertive communication. Set aside time when the two of you are alone to have these conversations. Then work on generating possible solutions and choose one you can both get behind.

Getting Ideas from Other Sources

Try settling disagreements by considering books, articles, podcasts, or the like that espouse the same approach to providing support as I'm advocating in this book. It's easy to find professionally written pieces about dealing with OCD in the family, as well as personal stories, online. You and your partner might grab one of these resources, read it (or watch it or listen to it) together, and then discuss your feelings about it. When you consider the new information as a team you foster an "us plus new information" position rather than a "me versus you" alignment.

10

Setting and Maintaining Expectations

If you're like most people I've worked with, you're inconsistent in how you respond to your relative's OCD. Sometimes you accommodate; other times you become angry or leave her to figure out how to manage anxiety on her own. Sometimes he gets away with poor conduct; at other times you come down hard on him for the same behavior. But responding inconsistently will keep you from achieving your goals of reducing the impact of OCD in your home. If, for example, your child can't predict how you'll respond when he becomes anxious, you can't expect him to understand that what you really want is for him to learn to manage anxiety on his own. And if you give in to your frustration and erupt in anger, you only escalate the level of hostility and squelch the voices of cooperation within him.

That's why you'll need to set clear and healthy expectations—and maintain them calmly and consistently. What really helps your family member become more confident and independent is knowing you'll always respond to him in the same, supportive way. Therefore, in this chapter you'll learn how to set and maintain supportive boundaries as a framework for reducing the negative effects of OCD in your household and relationships.

Setting Boundaries

Personal boundaries are guidelines for relationships. They are not actually walls between you and others as implied by the term, but rather connecting points. Boundaries define the behaviors, words, and interactions you're OK with and the ones you're *not* OK with and identify the consequences of crossing the boundary. Everyone has boundaries with other people, but those boundaries need to be healthy and clear if you're going to help your loved one and reduce OCD's grip on your family or relationship.

Healthy (Clear) Boundaries

The box below lists examples of healthy (or *clear*) boundaries. These are well-defined guidelines for acceptable and unacceptable interactions when it comes to OCD. If your child has OCD, healthy boundaries establish your role as a

---

Examples of Healthy (Clear) Boundaries

- I don't make decisions based on whether my child with OCD will become anxious or upset with me.
- I do not stand for being cursed at or threatened by my daughter.
- When Mom and Dad's bedroom door is closed, it means we want our privacy.
- I do not interrupt my work or social interactions because of my child's OCD.
- The car leaves for school at 7:45 no matter how anxious my son is feeling.
- I don't lie to other family members just to keep my wife from feeling anxious.
- Bedtimes and sleeping arrangements are not dictated by OCD or anxiety.
- All members of the household are expected to do their chores regardless of how anxious they're feeling.
- Everyone is responsible for flushing the toilet on their own when in the bathroom.
- My own emotions are not dictated by whether my husband is feeling anxious.
- My social plans are not put on hold because my daughter is feeling anxious.
- I do not tolerate loud noise in the house after bedtime.
- My ability to enjoy myself and be healthy is not affected by my son's OCD.
- I make sure there are appropriate consequences if my child violates my boundaries.

parent: you set examples, make the family rules, and use rewards and consequences fairly to shape good behavior. There's also a role for your child—even an older child living at home: follow your examples and be respectful of the rules. Depending on your child's age, healthy boundaries might also define acceptable communication patterns, such as how you speak to each other and what you share with (and ask of) each other. Since intimate relationships have greater equity than parent–child relationships, clear boundaries with your partner or spouse establish expectations for communication and openness, with less emphasis on making or following rules.

Clear boundaries also establish how you're unique from your loved one in healthy ways. They permit an appropriate degree of independence between you and your relative so that you have your own personal time and space. If you're the partner or spouse of someone with OCD, healthy boundaries create enough psychological space for you to have your own interests and friendships outside of your intimate partnership. They also allow you to have your own beliefs, thoughts, and feelings, which may or may not be the same as your partner's.

Healthy boundaries help you define yourself, as opposed to allowing your loved one's OCD to define you. They improve your self-image and protect you from being taken advantage of and feeling disrespected. You'll also have the space to provide feedback when your family member pushes your limits. In short, healthy boundaries allow you to support your loved one while also living your own life.

Healthy boundaries also benefit your loved one. They make interactions with you more predictable, which (especially for children) provides a sense of security. There's no mistaking what you expect, what constitutes a boundary violation, or the consequences of such a violation. This builds trust, better communication, greater self-assurance, and more independence for your loved one. With healthy boundaries, your relative will feel more capable of managing OCD when you begin to reduce your involvement—even if he initially pushes back.

Unhealthy (Blurry) Boundaries

In contrast, unhealthy or blurry boundaries erode expectations, confuse roles, and encourage unpredictable behavior, leading to the types of consequences listed in the box on the facing page. This leaves you feeling ineffective and easily exploited. It also leads to frustration and anger, impulsivity, and mutual blame.

The box on page 134 gives examples of blurry boundaries in the families

---

Consequences of Unhealthy Boundaries

- Too much of your daily life is dictated by a loved one's OCD.
- Your grown child with OCD has round-the-clock access to you either in person or electronically.
- Your personal time, space, or privacy has dwindled or disappeared because of OCD.
- Protecting your child from anxiety takes priority over work, family, or social activities.
- You do things for your family member that she should be doing for herself.
- You fall apart when your relative gets anxious or angry.
- Your loved one can easily get you to become angry or give in to OCD.
- You take your relative's anxiety-driven behavior personally (and perhaps retaliate).
- Your child can threaten violence (or act violently) without repercussions.
- Your adult grown child is living at home when he should be living independently.

---

and relationships of the four people you've been reading about in this book. Is it any wonder these families are stuck? Do you notice any blurred boundaries in your own family or relationship that might play a role in the accommodation patterns you identified in Chapter 8?

Blurred boundaries are common in families and relationships affected by OCD because OCD causes the person to doubt his ability to manage situations, responsibilities, anxiety, and obsessional thoughts. As a result, he grows more dependent on your protection. But it's a lot of work to resist your natural tendency to protect your loved one from distress. So you become more permissive and accommodating, especially if you believe too much anxiety is dangerous or that it's your job to be the protector. As a result, you become an extension of your loved one. It's as if OCD is now *your* problem as much as (if not more than) your relative's.

Can Boundaries Be Too Harsh?

Yes! Just as blurry boundaries are unhealthy, so too are limits that are overly rigid. They lead to becoming overly controlling or to keeping your relative

Examples of Unhealthy (Blurry) Boundaries

EDUARDO'S FAMILY

- Eduardo's mother's daily routine (including quitting her job) is dictated by OCD.
- Eduardo's mother does tasks for Eduardo that he is capable of doing on his own.
- Eduardo's mother puts up with threats and name-calling without there being any consequences for Eduardo.
- Eduardo dictates whether visitors are allowed inside the home and where they may sit.

ARIEL AND BEN

- Ben immediately drops what he's doing whenever Ariel asks him to help with rituals.
- Ben's social plans are dictated by Ariel's anxiety level.
- Ben's evening activities and bedtime are dictated by Ariel's need to do rituals.
- Ben puts up with Ariel yelling and cursing at him.

XAVIER AND HIS PARENTS

- Xavier is welcome to go into his parents' room unannounced at any time of day or night to get reassurance.
- Xavier's parents' vacation plans are dictated by Xavier's OCD.
- Xavier's mother constantly checks in with Xavier to make sure he's not angry with her.
- Xavier's parents give Xavier money for luxuries he wants (such as the latest electronic gadgets) to make him feel better and without expecting him to repay them or work on his own.

LINDA AND NICHOLAS

- The TV shows Nicholas watches and photos he displays are dictated by Linda's OCD.
- Nicholas's decisions about who he spends time with (his granddaughter, for example) are dictated by Linda's OCD.
- Nicholas's honesty with the rest of his family is dictated by Linda's OCD.

physically and emotionally distant. Here are some signs of overly rigid boundaries:

- You yell and scold your loved one for being disrespectful.
- You threaten or enact very severe punishments for even minor boundary violations.
- You don't attempt to have pleasant interactions with him.
- You dismiss your loved one and don't try to understand what she's going through.
- You expect your loved one to "just get over" her OCD.
- You avoid interactions with him and don't openly share your own thoughts or feelings.
- You're content being isolated and disconnected from your loved one.

Harsh boundaries come from feeling frustrated, taking your relative's problem personally, and showing no interest in understanding it better. They lead to violating your loved one's boundaries, which lowers her sense of security and self-esteem and negatively impacts her relationships. Just as with blurred boundaries, harsh ones are neither supportive of your relative with OCD nor effective in facilitating her independence and improvement.

Boundaries Are about You

If you look carefully at the examples in this chapter, you'll notice that boundaries are about deciding what *you* expect and what *you* will do; they're not about telling your loved one what to do. To illustrate, you can't keep your son from calling you from school in the middle of the day; but as the parent, you can take away his phone if he continues to call after being told to stop. Similarly, you can't stop your husband from calling and interrupting your workday just to ask for reassurance; but you can explain that you're busy and will call him back when it's more convenient, *but still not provide reassurance*. The take-home message here is that *you* determine your limits and boundaries.

Establishing Healthy Boundaries

Fifteen-year-old Anthony has morality obsessions about having accidentally broken an important rule—like unintentionally cheating on a test. He ritualizes by making daily confessions to the priest at his church. When his parents,

Ty and Rica, learned it was unhelpful to drop what they were doing and take Anthony to see the priest just to relieve anxiety, they set a boundary, letting him know that they would no longer allow OCD to disrupt their daily routine. At first, Anthony was anxious and upset. He would scream at his parents, "You don't love me anymore!" But Ty and Rica calmly explained the boundary they'd established: "Anthony, we understand you're upset with us, but we're no longer letting OCD interrupt our day. We're happy to play a board game with you when you've finished your homework, though." After a few days of sticking to this new boundary, Anthony caught on, and his screaming became a thing of the past.

As with Anthony's family, when you establish clear boundaries, you'll be both responsive to your loved one's needs, yet also maintain certain standards. You'll also set limits and be consistent in enforcing these boundaries. As a result, your relative will learn what to expect, become more self-reliant, and figure out that he's got to learn to manage OCD symptoms more independently. When your loved one's OCD becomes *his* problem—instead of yours—it will provide greater incentive to work with you or even seek professional help. So try the following:

Ask yourself why. The first step to clear boundaries is asking yourself why you need them in the first place. Take a look back at the Impact of OCD Rating Form from Chapter 8 and think about the ways OCD affects your relationships, family life, and personal welfare. How might blurred boundaries contribute to OCD's impact? How might *clearer* boundaries help you diminish OCD's impact?

Give yourself permission. You're entitled to choose what you'll put up with and what you won't. So trust yourself and don't let others define you. If you feel guilty that imposing boundaries will mean your family member has to face anxiety, remember that she's stronger and more resilient than it seems (for a reminder, see Chapter 6). Finally, don't let yourself believe that setting boundaries means you're *rejecting* your loved one; what you're rejecting is OCD!

Decide what you need. Look at the Identifying Accommodation Worksheet and Daily Accommodation Logs you completed in Chapter 8. Then review the examples of healthy and unhealthy boundaries in this chapter. What boundaries do you need to clarify so that there's more structure and support in your home to allow you to make changes? Consider the following types of boundaries:

- **Time.** Ty and Rica set a clear limit with Anthony about taking time away from other activities to respond to OCD. Ben decided he was going to bed when *he* got tired, rather than when Ariel decided that her nightly checking rituals were complete.

- **Personal space.** Ben decided he wasn't going to let Ariel's OCD keep him from an evening out with friends once a week. Xavier's parents decided their privacy was important: Xavier was no longer welcome in their bedroom if the door was closed.

- **Activities.** Eduardo's mother set the boundary that she was no longer going to clean Eduardo's room or make his bed. Nicholas hated being dishonest, so he decided he was no longer going to lie to his family about why Linda avoided certain activities.

- **Behavioral.** Eduardo's mother decided she wasn't going to put up with being yelled at, cursed at, or threatened by her son. To teach him to be more respectful, there would now be consequences for such behavior.

- **Emotional.** Ty and Rica decided it was OK if Anthony sometimes felt angry with them—they understood that effective parents do what's best in the long run for their children, even if it provokes short-term anger. Xavier's parents felt similarly and decided that their lives needed to be about things other than just protecting Xavier from distress.

Now it's your turn. Take some time to examine where clearer and more supportive boundaries can be set in your home and with your loved one. Then write them down in the form on page 139. Use the examples I've provided to guide you. In the next section, I'll cover how to preserve your boundaries using rewards and consequences.

Using Rewards to Clarify Boundaries and Encourage Appropriate Behavior

Eleven-year-old Hannah has obsessional fears that odd numbers will cause bad luck for her and her family. She insists that her mother, father, and older sister either avoid odd numbers or immediately say a special "good luck" phrase that Hannah devised as a ritual to prevent tragedy. When her family doesn't go along with these rules, Hannah throws tantrums and sometimes becomes aggressive until they give in.

Realizing that they care too much about Hannah to let things continue this way, her parents resolved to set clearer limits. They decided there would be no more avoidance and no more rituals; nor would they put up with tantrums, physical threats, or the destruction of property. But just because you set clear boundaries doesn't mean your relative must comply with them, so Hannah's parents needed a plan for encouraging their daughter to go along with the new boundaries. In this section, I'll cover how to properly use rewards to keep boundaries clear and encourage the behavior you want to see.

Catch Your Loved One Being Good

When you're frustrated with your family member's behavior, rewards may be the last thing on your mind. But people respond better to praise and recognition than to criticisms and corrections. That's why rewarding good behavior, or what psychologists call *positive reinforcement,* is such an effective behavior modification technique. If you provide rewards when your relative respects your boundaries or appropriately manages anxiety and OCD, she'll learn to do more of these things because she likes the good feelings that come with receiving praise . . . not to mention the actual reward itself. And while material rewards like games or money often work perfectly well, social rewards like praise ("You handled that situation very well; I know how difficult that was"), affection (such as hugs, kisses, a high five, or an arm around the shoulder), and other forms of genuine positive attention can be even *more* effective.

The other perk of using rewards is that you never have to force your relative to change her behavior. You're simply creating an incentive for her to behave appropriately. Of course, the particular behaviors you'll want to reward will be specific to your family member's obsessions, compulsions, age, maturity level, and relationship to you. Here are some suggestions:

- **For children:** Facing a feared situation, resisting a ritual, playing quietly, cooperating with a sibling, completing chores independently, putting in a lot of effort on a difficult task, being on time, trying something new

- **For an older son or daughter:** Facing a fear, resisting a ritual, cooperating with parents, studying for school, completing household chores, applying for jobs, behaving maturely, making good decisions, becoming independent, managing difficult situations, being on time

- **For a partner or spouse:** Facing a fear, resisting rituals, spending time together free from interference by OCD, managing OCD situations independently, communicating effectively, cooperating, demonstrating affection, trying something new

Healthy Boundaries I Want to Establish

Time:

Personal space:

Activities:

Behavioral:

Emotional:

From *The Family Guide to Getting Over OCD* by Jonathan S. Abramowitz. Copyright © 2021 The Guilford Press. Purchasers of this book can photocopy and/or download enlarged versions of this material (see the box at the end of the Contents).

Making Rewards Work

For rewards to work, they have to create enough of an incentive for your family member to change his behavior. Here are some tips for making sure you've got an effective reward system in place.

- Use rewards your loved one really wants or enjoys. Think about hobbies, interests, pastimes, and other things she values.

- Consider social rewards for children and adults. Privileges (like staying up late to watch the big game), affection, and spending one-on-one time can be just as gratifying as material rewards; and they're easier and less costly (or even free) to give your relative.

- Keep a written list of potential rewards (and an ear out for what you can add to the list) so you're never stuck trying to think of something on the fly.

- Help your family member make the connection between behaving appropriately and receiving rewards by explaining what he's got to do (or not do) to earn them. Draw up a written plan (especially for a younger child) if necessary.

- Give the reward as soon as possible after you catch your family member doing something good and tell her what you liked about her behavior and why she's earned the reward (for example, "Ariel, you didn't ask me to check tonight, and I'm very proud of you. How about we cuddle up and watch a few episodes of your favorite show?").

- Let your relative know that you want her to succeed.

- Reward *effort* when the outcome isn't under your loved one's direct control. For example, reward *applying* for jobs since he can't control whether he's actually hired.

- Make sure the reward matches the achievement: smaller prizes for less challenging accomplishments and bigger ones for more significant breakthroughs.

- If you promise a reward, make sure your loved one receives it.

- Make sure your loved one actually does what you require before getting the reward.

- Never take away rewards that have already been earned.

But Rewards Don't Work for My Relative!

Have you tried rewarding good behavior only to find that this approach doesn't seem to work for your loved one? Here are some common concerns and tips to try out before totally giving up on rewards:

"I can't get him to change." If you've said this to yourself, you might be misusing rewards as *bribes,* which is not how they're meant to be used. Bribes involve giving your family member something so he'll promise to change his behavior right then and there ("I'll buy you a candy bar if you stop asking me for reassurance"). But any success you have will be short-lived. Rewards, on the other hand, are given only *after* he exhibits appropriate behavior ("If you don't ask me for reassurance today, I'll let you pick out a treat at the store after dinner"). What's the difference? Rewards help your relative change over the long run by teaching him that privileges and incentives have to be earned with good behavior.

Are you rewarding the wrong behavior? It's easy to overlook that simply getting attention can be a strong reward. So, if your loved one's getting attention for being anxious, doing rituals, or violating boundaries, rewards *are* working—it just that the wrong behavior is being rewarded!

Take 16-year-old Matthew, who did extensive repeating rituals—stepping back and forth, flicking a light switch—whenever repugnant thoughts (such as "What if I killed my cat?") came to mind. These rituals were keeping Matthew from getting to school, but when I suggested rewards for better attendance, Matthew's mother was dismissive and told me that rewards never worked for her son. Interestingly, an hour after our session I found Matthew and his mother still stuck in the hallway outside my office. Matthew was ritualizing, and his mother was standing beside him waiting patiently. When I suggested she head out to the car and tell Matthew she was leaving, she said she needed to stay with him. Then she gave Matthew big a hug and told him, "Mommy would never leave you." Indeed, rewards *did* work for Matthew! Unfortunately, Mom was rewarding the rituals by giving Matthew attention and allowing him to miss school.

"She doesn't do *anything* good." Of course she does; it's just that her boundary-breaking and OCD-related behavior is what really grabs your attention (she yells, interrupts, or does rituals). On the other hand, when she's behaving appropriately it's less obvious (remaining calm, being independent, *not* asking for reassurance). Try to actively catch her in these moments and reward her. You can also look for positives within annoying situations. Your daughter is still taking 45-minute showers, but they *were* 90 minutes. Rewarding this accomplishment can motivate her to continue reducing the length of her showering rituals.

"She doesn't care about getting material rewards." Fine. But whether she admits it or not, she wants your attention. So don't underestimate the power of a high five, a hug, or telling her how proud you are of what she did. Sometimes the best reward is just being recognized for doing something well.

"He doesn't care about *anything.*" Don't fall into this trap—of course he does. But maybe he's satisfied with what he already has. Eduardo was content to stay in his room all day because he had his computer and gaming system there for entertainment. If your son already enjoys lots of comforts and luxuries, there might not be much incentive to respond to your rewards. But this doesn't mean he doesn't care. Try creating more incentive by removing something he takes for granted (for example, by password-protecting a computer or restricting the use of the car) and use this as a reward to be earned back with appropriate behavior.

Using Consequences to Clarify Boundaries and Discourage Inappropriate Behavior

Consequences are negative outcomes that result from a person's behavior. When an action is followed by something unpleasant, that action is less likely to occur in the future. As you'll learn in this section, there are two types of consequences: *natural* and *logical*. Both help clarify boundaries and teach your loved one to become more self-sufficient and aware of her decisions.

Natural Consequences

Natural consequences are negative outcomes that you don't plan or deliver—they just happen organically, as a matter of course. Eduardo breaks his phone during a tantrum, so he no longer has a phone to use. Ariel drove back and forth five times to recheck the front door, so she gets reprimanded for being late to work. The natural consequences of having OCD may include painful feelings and emotions, such as anxiety and embarrassment; consequences imposed by society, such as problems in school or at work; and consequences inflicted by the forces of nature, such as sore hands from excessive washing.

Finally, natural consequences can result from your enforcing boundaries. For example, your daughter runs out of clean clothes because you refuse to do her laundry "the OCD way." Here are some other examples:

- Your son with a fear of ticks has to miss out on playing soccer with his friends because he avoids grassy areas.
- Your husband stays up late doing rituals, so he's overly tired the next day at work.
- Your adult daughter can't buy what she wants since OCD keeps her from maintaining a job and earning money.

These consequences sound pretty bad, and maybe you've been protecting your loved one from them. But they're actually your ally because they provide incentive for your relative to work toward reducing OCD's effects. Of course, it's difficult to just let someone you love face the unpleasant effects of OCD head-on. That's why I'll show you how to use natural consequences in a compassionate and supportive way that pushes your family member to take responsibility for managing OCD (or get professional help) so she can avoid future pain and be happier and more independent down the road. Read on.

Don't get in the way! If you swoop in to save the day, natural consequences can't work. If Eduardo's mother buys him a new phone, he'll never learn to curb his tantrums. On the other hand, not having a phone (or having to pay for a replacement) would be a constant reminder to better control himself. Similarly, if Ben calls the school where Ariel teaches and makes excuses for her lateness, he keeps Ariel from realizing the urgency of getting help to stop her excessive checking rituals.

Stand firm. Impose your limits as part of the natural consequences. That is, don't allow your boundaries to blur to make things easier for your loved one. If you've established the boundary that you're not flushing the toilet for your daughter (a good boundary to have!), then she's got to learn to manage her fear of germs within this limit: the bathroom will stink unless she flushes. If you've decided you're not giving your adult son money until he begins applying for jobs, then not having spending money becomes a natural consequence of refusing to apply.

Show plenty of compassion. Let your relative know you understand what he's going through and that you wish things were different; and convey optimism he'll figure out a better way to handle the situation next time (but don't directly tell him what to do). For example, "It must be awful having to put up with that horrible smell in your bathroom. But I'm sure you'll figure out how to handle it." Avoid lecturing, scolding, or saying "I told you so." And don't do anything to add more shame, blame, or pain.

Safety first! Never allow natural consequences to place your loved one in real physical danger, for example, if she's gone days on end without eating. Missing a few meals won't cause harm, but if it's been several days, you might intervene and seek medical attention. Remember, though, that anxiety, panic, and other forms of emotional distress do *not* pose actual physical risks; and neither does missing out on social events or having trouble at school or work. If you're not sure whether a natural consequence would be too dangerous or detrimental, it's best to consult an advocate or professional. You can use logical consequences in place of natural ones if need be.

What if there are no unpleasant natural consequences? Even with these rules of thumb in place, there might be times when your loved one accepts the consequences of her OCD-related behavior and sees them as "no big deal." Ultimately, her behavior is up to her—which can be a hard fact to accept. Here again, your backup plan is to use logical consequences to help your relative learn what is and is not appropriate.

Logical Consequences

Logical consequences involve taking action when boundaries are crossed. For example, if Eduardo curses at his parents, they might take away his computer for an entire day so he'll learn not to cross this boundary. Since logical consequences give one person power over another, they're not appropriate for relationships built on equality, such as with an intimate partner. But this strategy can be effective with children of any age (including adults) if they're living in your home and dependent on you. Here's how to use logical consequences with your son or daughter.

Take away items and privileges. If you decide you need to punish a behavior—perhaps your family member is damaging property, causing harm, or being disrespectful in ways you simply can't ignore—use your role as a parent to take away privileges and other things he values, such as favorite toys, clothes, electronic devices, car privileges, or allowance money. I've worked with parents who changed the Wi-Fi password and removed TVs and game consoles from their child's bedroom. It's your home, and as a parent you have the right to take these things away to support your child by teaching him that certain behavior is not acceptable. Just make sure what you're taking away is a *luxury* and not a *necessity*. Don't, for example, take away piano time if your daughter plays to manage anxiety or the car your son needs to get to work. I recommend keeping a list of items and privileges you can easily take away should punishment be required.

Keep calm and don't overdo it. When you're really upset with your family member, it's easy to go in with guns blazing and threaten extreme consequences. But remember that all that attention can be rewarding. So give logical consequences without much fanfare. Calmly provide a *brief* explanation of why your relative is being punished and then move on without getting dragged into arguments or power struggles (for example, "You are not allowed to use the car tonight because you interrupted my telephone conversation five times"). And consequences don't need to be excessive. Stick with those you can easily administer so that you don't make too much work for yourself. And, of course, never use physical punishment, shaming, or humiliation.

Give warnings and always follow through. Logical consequences work best when your loved one learns the connection between the behavior and the consequences. So clearly let her know when she's pushing your limits and that there will be negative consequences if she doesn't change her behavior. Also, make sure it's understood that your problem is with what she *did*, not with her as a *person*. Finally, resist the urge to let your relative off the hook once you've promised a negative consequence—even if she goes and changes her behavior. You won't be taken seriously, and your boundaries will become blurred. You can explain by saying, "There still needs to be consequences for what happened earlier, but I'm very proud of you for changing your behavior."

Pick your battles. You don't have to respond to *every* boundary violation, so sometimes it's better just to ignore bad behavior—especially if your child is purposely committing boundary violations to get your attention. In fact, when your loved one's behavior isn't destructive or dangerous, ignoring it is the ideal response because it minimizes attention seeking. Remember Hannah from page 137? When she started her tantrums, her parents calmly walked away and left her to calm down on her own (going into their room and closing the door if necessary). Only later would they praise her for soothing herself. After a while, Hannah got it. She learned that tantrums wouldn't help her get her way or her parents' attention. What behaviors could you begin ignoring?

Consistency: The Key to Success

Being *consistent* means following through and doing as you say you will. Your family member with OCD might not be happy with the changes you're making—establishing boundaries, rewarding only the good behavior, and making sure inappropriate behavior has consequences. But when you respond in the same way time after time, she'll learn what to expect from you. And she'll be able to predict how you (and others) will react. This doesn't mean she won't test you to see if you'll give in. But if you're consistent in how you respond, she'll eventually learn that certain outcomes follow certain behaviors, and she'll begin to problem-solve on her own and make better choices. This is especially true for children, who develop self-confidence and learn to understand the world through consistency.

Think of yourself as a slot machine in a casino. Then picture your relative with OCD as a hopeful gambler putting money in the machine and pulling the lever, eager to win the jackpot. If your boundaries are blurry and you've responded to OCD inconsistently in the past—sometimes you accommodate, sometimes you don't—your loved one knows there's a chance you'll let bad behavior go, protect him from anxiety, or help with rituals. In other words, there's a chance he'll win the jackpot. This is what psychologists call the principle of "variable ratio reinforcement," and it's why gamblers have difficulty tearing themselves away from casinos. If you're not consistent in how you respond to your relative's behavior, you're basically training him to keep playing the slot machine—which is you!

To make matters worse, when you're inconsistent you undermine your authority by saying one thing and doing another. If you say, "We're not going to wait for you to finish your rituals" but then fail to back this up with your actions and wait 30 minutes to leave for a family outing while your son performs compulsions over and over, he gets the message that you don't really mean what you say, and it starts to lose its meaning.

Why is it so hard to be consistent? Being consistent is time-consuming and requires planning, patience, and perseverance. But sometimes it's just easier to do what seems most convenient in the moment. Nicholas, for example, was frustrated that Linda kept asking for assurance that she wasn't a pedophile. Yet after vowing not to give her any more reassurance, he would sometimes get so fed up that it was just easier to answer her questions.

The belief that "too much" anxiety will harm your loved one can also make it more difficult to be consistent. You learned in Chapter 6, however, that even intense anxiety, obsessions, and uncertainty are safe and temporary and therefore do not require deviating from your plan to withhold rewards or deliver negative consequences. Let the temporary distress become an incentive for your family member to change her behavior.

Finally, it's difficult to be consistent when your loved one is pushing back. Depending on factors such as age, maturity, social skills, and creativity, this pushback might take the form of objections such as "I hate you!" or "You don't love me!" or of pleading, arguing, or negotiating. He might resist or pretend he doesn't hear you. She might become angrier and more emotional. Aggressive behavior isn't out of the question either. But pushback is normal. It comes from a place of fear (not true hate). To your loved one, obsessions seem like real threats that she has to deal with to avoid disaster. So don't take it personally; it's your relative's way of saying, "Wait a minute, I don't like what's going on here!" In Chapter 12, you'll learn effective strategies for remaining consistent in the face of such pushback.

How can you be more consistent? One way to maintain consistency is to review the material covered in Part II of this book on keeping your stress levels in check (Chapter 5), recognizing anxiety as safe and manageable (Chapter 6), and communicating effectively (Chapter 7). You can also review the information in *this* chapter on boundaries, rewards, and consequences and discuss it with one or more family advocates. Armed with all of this knowledge and support, you're ready to begin making changes. In the next chapter, I'll help you develop a plan for reducing accommodation and begin putting it into practice.

11

Reducing Accommodation

Now that you've informed your loved one of what's to come and prepared yourself with healthy boundaries, you're ready to set specific accommodation reduction goals and get to work. We'll begin by setting goals for reducing accommodation—and making sure they're the kinds of goals you're likely to achieve. I'll give you loads of suggestions, as well as examples of how to reduce accommodation for different types of OCD symptoms. I'll also give you strategies to help you effectively and consistently implement your plan, including what to say to your relative when you refuse to comply with OCD's rules. Often this process goes smoothly. Yet it's important to be prepared in case your loved one becomes confrontational, from arguing with you (most common) to making threats or engaging in more seriously disruptive and harmful behavior (less common). That's why I've dedicated Chapter 12 to helping you deal with different forms of pushback. *If you anticipate any type or level of resistance when you begin reducing accommodation, I suggest reading Chapter 12 immediately after finishing this one so that you're prepared before you begin implementing any changes.*

Setting Accommodation Reduction Goals

The process of reducing accommodation begins with setting goals for yourself. Goals give you something to work toward and keep you focused through thick and thin. The Accommodation Reduction Goals form on the facing page provides space for listing goals you want to achieve. But before you begin writing, let me recommend using the acronym SMART to help you optimize your goals and maximize your likelihood of success. While this acronym

Accommodation Reduction Goals

Order	Goal

From *The Family Guide to Getting Over OCD* by Jonathan S. Abramowitz. Copyright © 2021 The Guilford Press. Purchasers of this book can photocopy and/or download enlarged versions of this material (see the box at the end of the Contents).

comes from the corporate world, it applies equally well to setting goals in your personal life. Specifically, your goals should be:

S = Specific

M = Measurable

A = Achievable

R = Relevant

T = Time bound

Specific. Make your goals as detailed and specific as possible. Stipulate exactly what you want to achieve. This will help you focus your efforts and clearly define what you're striving to do. Simply saying "My goal is to stop accommodating" is too hazy. Instead, use "I will no longer help Ariel check the doors and appliances before bed."

As the box on the facing page shows, specific goals can fall into two categories. The goals shown on the left side of the table depend on other people, such as your loved one, agreeing with you and doing what you want them to do. For example, getting your husband to stop texting you for reassurance depends on his deciding not to send you texts. Similarly, having your daughter get a job depends not only on her behavior (submitting an application) but also on employers and the pool of other job applicants. On the other hand, look at the goals on the right side. Do they require your loved one to cooperate? The answer is no. Achieving these goals rests solely on your own actions. Because you've got a better chance of meeting goals when they're fully under your control, these are the kinds of goals you'll want to set. Keep the focus on changing *your own* behavior.

Measurable. Your goals for reducing accommodation also need to be measurable so that you know when you've succeeded. So choose concrete goals you can easily keep track of. The goals listed in the box all adhere to this rule. "Stop answering Antonio's texts" provides a specific target to be measured: whether or not you've responded to your son's texts. On the other hand, "Do a better job of not accommodating Antonio's OCD" is not measurable: How will you decide if you've done a *better* job? Setting goals to change observable behaviors (that someone else would be able to see) is your best bet for making sure your goals are measurable.

Achievable. Your goals should challenge you to stay focused and committed to your program, but at the same time they need to be realistic. If you

Types of Goals	
Goals that depend on others	**Goals that depend only on you**
• Antonio will stop texting me to ask for reassurance all day long	• I will stop answering Antonio's texts
• Annie will get a job	• We will stop paying for Annie if she's not earning money for herself
• Brandon will take a shorter shower so he doesn't make us late for church	• We will leave for church without Brandon if he's not ready when it's time to go
• Harrison will limit his time playing video games	• I'll take Harrison's video games away
• Shira will start driving again	• I won't drive Shira around or run errands for her
• Jake will allow people to sit in his chair	• We will allow anyone to sit on any piece of furniture in the house

set goals that stretch you (and your loved one with OCD) somewhat, you will continue to put in the effort to achieve them. On the other hand, you probably won't stay committed to goals that are too far out of reach. For example, "I will never again reassure Antonio" is probably unattainable, especially if you've become accustomed to providing reassurance and your son is clever about getting it from you. Instead, "I will stop answering Antonio's texts when he asks for reassurance" is probably a more reasonable (and also a more *specific*) goal. Don't bite off more than you can chew! And of course, be careful not to set goals too low or you'll feel like you're not making progress.

Relevant. Without an emotional tie to your goals, you'll lose the motivation to stick with them. In this case, they should obviously relate to (1) helping your loved one develop self-confidence and the ability to manage anxiety on her own, (2) reducing your involvement in her OCD symptoms, and (3) improving your and your family's quality of life. Tying goals to one or more of these things will build your commitment to success.

To ensure that your goals are relevant, review your responses on the

Impact of OCD Rating Form (pages 103–104) and think about the areas of life that OCD affects the most. What problems need to be addressed because they're hindering your own health and well-being or that of your family or relationship? Then examine the Identifying Accommodation Worksheet and Daily Accommodation Logs you completed in Chapter 8 and look for patterns of accommodation that you'd need to end to address these issues and reduce OCD's impact. In what situations do you find yourself accommodating your loved one? Eduardo's mother, for example, was running herself ragged taking care of her son, so she decided that she needed to stop getting up extra early to clean the bathroom for Eduardo. This goal would give her an extra hour or two of sleep, which she greatly needed. It would also support Eduardo by pushing him to manage his fear of germs on his own each morning.

You can also use the worksheets and logs to identify accommodation patterns that appear frequently or with regularity, as well as those associated with financial, social, and time costs. A father I worked with set the goal of no longer paying for his 35-year-old son's Internet access. His son, who had an obsessional fear that he was developing amyotrophic lateral sclerosis (ALS or Lou Gehrig's disease), was living at home and refusing to find employment (or help for his OCD) because he wanted to spend his time checking the Internet for information that would help him determine whether he was really developing this very serious (and rare) disease.

Time bound. Finally, your goals should have a time frame. This means stipulating when you'll begin changing your behavior—for example, "beginning tomorrow." By specifying a time frame, you make your goal a priority, which increases motivation. Goals without specific time frames are less likely to be met because you feel you can put them off.

What Are *Your* Goals?

Now take some time to think through what accommodation behaviors you'd like to target. In what specific situations are you likely to try to protect your loved one from OCD symptoms or anxiety? Which accommodation patterns interfere with your relationships or routines, or involve going to extremes? Which ones come up frequently or take up a great deal of time and lead to feeling dissatisfied with family or relationship life? And which seem to prevent your loved one from learning that experiences such as anxiety, unwanted thoughts, and uncertainty are safe and manageable? Ending these patterns should be your accommodation reduction goals. Write them down on the

Accommodation Reduction Goals worksheet (on page 149) and make sure they adhere to the SMART criteria you just read. The worksheet contains spaces for 15 goals, but you might have more or fewer, and you can list them in any order. The next section provides ideas for how to reduce accommodation for different types of symptoms. Use these as you consider setting your goals.

Once you've got your list, rank your goals from first to last by priority and the sequence in which you plan to address them (using the "Order" column). Which accommodation behaviors get in the way the most, take up the greatest amount of time or occur most frequently, create the most frustration, or prove costliest? Maybe you'll begin with these if you want to see big differences right away. Or you could plan to go more gradually, beginning with reducing those accommodation patterns that seem like they'll be easiest to address and working up to more challenging ones over time. There's no right or wrong approach, and your rankings aren't etched in stone. The purpose is to have a road map for moving from goal to goal. Once you get started, you'll periodically want to evaluate your progress with these goals. So be sure to read pages 181–184 at the beginning of Chapter 13, where I've covered how to do this.

Accommodation Reduction Goals for Different Types of OCD Symptoms

There are countless varieties of obsessions and compulsions, as well as ways to accommodate these symptoms. In view of this, and to help you set your own goals, here are ideas and examples of accommodation reduction goals for different types of obsessional fears, avoidance behaviors, and compulsive rituals (as well as some ideas that apply more generally across the different forms of OCD). I've tried to be as comprehensive and inclusive as possible so that you'll find some suggestions that apply to you and your relative—though you'll likely need to improvise to some extent since your relative's OCD symptoms, and the patterns of accommodation that occur in your family or relationship, may be unique to your particular situation. As challenging as these goals might seem, remember that you are working to help your loved one become more self-confident and independent in the face of OCD.

Contamination Obsessions and Decontamination Compulsions

- Refuse to wash your hands because of a family member's OCD
- Refuse to wash your hands, clean items or rooms, or pick things up off the floor because of OCD

- Refuse to change clothes or take extra showers because of OCD

- Refuse to do extra laundry (or to do *any* laundry for an adult with OCD)

- End special food preparation routines related to OCD

- Refrain from buying special cleaning supplies (or refuse to provide money to buy them)

- Refuse to supply antibacterial hand sanitizers (or to use them yourself)

- Refuse to wait, or make excuses for lateness, because of washing or cleaning rituals

- Refuse to open doors, flush toilets, or handle "contaminated" items for your loved one

- Allow guests to enter your home if you wish to invite them

- Refuse to obey OCD rules for avoiding places or objects inside or outside your home

- Refuse to wipe down items before bringing them into the home

- Use household chemicals as needed and as directed by the packaging

- Do not refrain from any behaviors that your loved one fears would spread contamination (such as giving hugs, sharing food, sharing clothes, and the like) unless there is an actual medical reason for doing so (such as if someone is truly sick)

Obsessions about Responsibility for Harm and Compulsive Checking

- Refrain from checking things *with* or *for* your loved one

- Refuse to watch your relative check

- Refuse to wait for your relative or provide excuses for lateness because of checking rituals

- Reduce how much responsibility you assume in anxiety-provoking situations

- Refuse to drive for your loved one with obsessions about accidents or "hit-and-runs"

- Refuse to do paperwork for your loved one

Reassurance–Seeking Rituals

- Refuse to offer assurances to your loved one
- Refuse to help your loved one analyze or remember things related to obsessional doubts
- It's OK to provide reality checks if your loved one sincerely doesn't know and is willing to accept a "yes" or "no" answer; but avoid answering the same questions repeatedly and do not try to answer detailed questions that are meant to attain guarantees
- Let your relative know you're sorry he's anxious, but that you can't answer reassurance-seeking questions any longer
- Respond by saying something neutral, such as "that's an interesting idea"
- Respond to excessive apologies, explaining, or confessing with silence, by walking away, or by pretending you can't understand your loved one
- Refuse to assist with Internet searches about obsessional fears (consider denying your loved one access to the Internet if searching for assurance is a problem)
- Refuse to search the Bible with (or for) your loved one for reassurance
- Refuse to help your loved one seek reassurance from others (such as experts or religious authorities)

Obsessions about Sex, Harm, Violence, or Religion

- Refuse to go out of your way to avoid stimuli that prompt obsessional thoughts
- Refuse to refrain from mentioning or discussing topics, words, or other stimuli that provoke obsessional thoughts
- Refuse to hide or dispose of items that provoke obsessions
- Refuse to handle knives (or other sharp objects) for your loved one
- Refuse to avoid movies, shows, or other stimuli or situations that provoke obsessions
- Refuse to repeat religious rituals or ceremonies because of OCD
- Refuse to repeat prayers because of OCD
- Do not distract your loved one or help her think positive thoughts

Mental Rituals

- Do not help your loved one remember, analyze, or review events or situations

- Don't wait for your loved one to complete mental rituals

- Don't ask about or respond with interest to your loved one's mental rituals

Incompleteness Obsessions and Ordering/Arranging Rituals

- Refuse to help put or keep items in their "proper" order, place, or arrangement

- Refuse to help with "balancing" or "evening" things out

- Refuse to keep things arranged a certain way because of OCD

- Refrain from waiting for your family member to complete rituals

General Goal Suggestions

- Stop doing _____ if it protects your loved one from obsessional thoughts or anxiety

- Return to usual schedules and routines if they've been disrupted or rearranged by OCD

- Return to usual sleeping arrangements and bedtimes

- Return to usual eating and mealtime patterns

- Refuse to reschedule, modify, or terminate individual or family plans because of OCD

- Refuse to help with household chores or responsibilities because of OCD

- Refuse to accompany or supervise your relative because of OCD

- Do what's most convenient for you or the family regardless of any rules that OCD has set

- Refuse to wait for your loved one to finish rituals or allow him to slow you down

- Refuse to let your loved one rush you because of OCD

- Refuse to make decisions and excuses for your loved one

- Accept invitations to (and attend) social engagements even if they create anxiety

- Refrain from walking on eggshells around your loved one with OCD

- Remove any incentives (such as video games) for your loved one to stay home or stay in his room because of OCD

- Refrain from giving your relative any money that could be used for avoidance or rituals

- Suggest that others in the family stop their accommodation behaviors as well

- Don't ask your relative about, or bring up the topic of, her OCD symptoms

As examples of how to personalize your accommodation reduction goals, here are partial goal lists from the families of the four individuals we've been following throughout this book (later in the chapter you'll see their complete plans):

Eduardo's Mother's Goals

- Stop taking food to Eduardo's bedroom

- Stop making Eduardo's bed and cleaning his room

- Clean the bathroom only during routine housecleaning (once per week) instead of every day

- Allow people to sit or go where they want in the house

Ben's Goals

- Stop helping with Ariel's checking and reassurance-seeking rituals at night

- No longer leave work to do checking for Ariel during the day

- Stop responding to Ariel's texts asking for reassurance

- Refuse to call Ariel's employer to explain why she's late or absent

Xavier's Parents' Goals

- Stop trying to reassure Xavier that he hasn't sinned

- Take Xavier off the payroll at the family business (hardware store)

- Stop listening to Xavier's repeated confessions
- Observe our faith the way we want, not according to Xavier's demands

Nicholas's Goals

- Invite Emma's parents to bring Emma to our house
- Stop making excuses for why Linda is avoiding Emma
- Stop reassuring Linda that she's not a pedophile
- Watch my favorite TV shows even if Linda is at home
- Hang up pictures of Emma around the house

Plan to Chip Away at Accommodation

Rather than trying to tackle every goal at once, I recommend phasing out accommodation patterns in a gradual way (I'll show you examples a bit later in this chapter). One strategy that works for many families is to end one accommodation pattern each week, building on previous weeks and making sure that old patterns don't creep back in. Of course, how quickly you pull yourself (and others) out of accommodating is up to you; there's no one right way to do it.

Why not end accommodation behaviors all at once? For one thing, you're more likely to have long-term success with reducing accommodation (as with any goal) when you make changes in gradual steps. I've seen many overly eager parents and partners try to stop all their accommodation at the same time, only to find that they end up accomplishing none of their goals. Second, your relative will be able to prepare for and adjust to the changes you're making much more easily when you make them little by little as opposed to all at once. And succeeding in one area will help motivate her to work hard in other areas—perhaps without you even having to say or do anything. If you feel that progress is slower than you'd hoped for, try using the stress management skills in Chapter 5 to keep you feeling optimistic about moving forward.

What should you do about the other accommodation behaviors while you're chipping away at them one at a time? For now, continue doing what you've been doing, but avoid arguing about it with your loved one. Instead, remind yourself that this is a process and stay focused on the changes you *are* making. Even small adjustments help your loved one learn the extremely valuable message that he is stronger than he thinks and that he can get better. Think about it this way: if it takes you 15 minutes to run 1 mile, but you want to be able to run it in 8 minutes, you wouldn't expect to cut your time down all at once (this would be next to impossible and set you up for failure). Instead, you would gradually build your skills and your confidence by first aiming for 14 minutes, then for 13, 12, and so on until you could run the mile in 8 minutes. In the same vein, it's important to set up your program to maximize the chances of success for your relative. When he makes these adjustments, it will lead to more confidence for him and greater satisfaction for you.

Preemptive Troubleshooting: Think It Through

Before you get going, you'll want to do some planning to make sure you've worked out all the kinks in your plan. So take the time to sit down (perhaps with a partner or advocate) and really think through the first change you're planning to make . . . *and how it could go wrong*. This will help you avoid some of the challenges you anticipate facing and allow things to go more smoothly when you implement your plan. You'll do this each time a change is made to the accommodation routine. Here are examples of the kinds of questions to ask yourself:

- What could come up that would keep me from carrying out my plan?
- In what situations might it be tricky to refuse to accommodate?
- Are there things my relative might say or do (or not do) that would persuade me to give in?
- Are there situations where I might feel too uncomfortable or embarrassed dealing with my loved one in front of others?
- Will there be situations when I'm pressed for time and might end up giving in?
- Are there things my loved one could do in response that would be unacceptable to me?

Next, think through possible solutions to these potential obstacles. What will you do if they arise? I suggest writing down your ideas and solutions so you'll have them available if and when the time comes. In Chapter 12, I'll give you recommendations for how to manage situations in which your relative becomes argumentative, hostile, or aggressive. And if you're concerned about this level of pushback, I suggest reading ahead before implementing your plan.

Nicholas, for example, thought through how he'd handle situations in which Linda's obsessions were triggered in public. When this happened in the past, Linda would become emotional and Nicholas would immediately calm her down to avoid any humiliation. But after learning (in Chapter 10) that natural (unpleasant) consequences are a powerful form of behavioral modification, Nicholas decided he would let his wife work through the distress on her own from now on (for example, by letting Linda know where he would be waiting for her when she felt better). As awkward as this felt, Nicholas knew it would help Linda learn how to better manage her obsessions next time. Similarly, Eduardo's parents considered what they would do if their son became unruly or even violent when accommodation was withheld. They jointly developed a plan (which you'll read about in the next chapter) for how to prevent such behavior from interfering with their accommodation reduction strategies.

Putting Your Plan into Action

Notifying Your Loved One

Now that you've settled on a plan, it's time to get started! The first thing you'll do is prepare your loved one for the first change (or changes) you'll be making. With each successive change, you'll give your relative a similar notification. You can think of these notifications as similar to the overall declaration you made in Chapter 9, just more specific in their focus. And you can use the same suggestions to help you craft and deliver these messages each time you're ready to work on a new goal. Remember to include the following points in each announcement:

- You appreciate the difficulty your relative is going through.

- You're changing how you respond to OCD because you love your family member and you're determined to help her get better.

- You're confident in her ability to cope with the changes you've planned and with the anxiety she'll probably experience.

- You'd like to work on this together as a team; but that's *her* choice. You're sticking with your plans for making changes either way.

As an example, Brittany, the 11-year-old girl with tapping rituals you read about in Chapter 9, was watching TV by herself when her parents approached her and explained the new changes they would be making as follows:

"Brittany, as you know from our talk several days ago, Mom and I have been thinking about how we can all work together to help you get better at managing OCD. We know how hard it is for you to stop your tapping rituals because you're afraid it will cause bad luck to our family. But we also know that things would be OK even if you didn't do these rituals and that you're strong and can handle the anxious feelings. So we've decided that we're not going to wait for rituals anymore when it's time to leave the house. The car will leave at the scheduled time. You're 11 years old now, and we know you'll be fine staying home by yourself for a few hours if you can't get ready in time. If you would like, we'll even give you some warning time because we hope you'll join us instead of getting stuck tapping—but that will be your choice. We know this new rule will take some getting used to, but changing how we all deal with OCD will help you so that rituals don't interfere with family outings anymore. We love you, we know you're strong, and it's our job to help you get better."

Since Brittany had been cooperative during the initial declaration, her parents presented this plan as an opportunity to work together. Notice that Brittany was even included in planning the process (she could ask for warning time to get prepared). Giving your relative—especially if she is younger—a say (even if it's a minor detail) builds motivation to join forces and helps prevent conflict. Yet as with the original declaration, it's important to avoid engaging in debates over your plan with your relative.

On the other hand, if you anticipate significant pushback, prepare a written message (as I described in Chapter 9) that you can leave with your relative and then begin making your changes (you'll want to read Chapter 12 before getting started). Sample accommodation reduction plans for Eduardo, Ariel, Xavier, and Linda, as well as the script each family used when introducing the first change they planned to make, appear a bit later in this chapter.

Consistency, Again!

In Chapter 10 you read about the importance of consistency when using rewards and consequences, and it's just as crucial with reducing accommodation. So, indulge me in a quick pep talk: If you're going to get untangled from OCD, help your loved one become more independent, and improve the environment in your household, you've got to implement your plan so that your loved one knows what to expect from you. There will be times when sticking with your plan is exhausting, frustrating, and time-consuming. And if you're feeling anxious, frustrated, tired, or in a hurry, it will seem easier to just let things slide. But don't let convenience win out over consistency. Consider your hard work an investment in your loved one's self-confidence and improvement, in your family's quality of life, and in your own independence from OCD. Think carefully about possible barriers to consistency and make sure to address them—perhaps with the help of a partner or spouse (if you're the parent of someone with OCD) or an outside advocate.

With this pep talk in mind, you're ready to put your plan into practice. As you think about how you'll reduce accommodation, use the following examples of goals and notifications to guide your planning and implementation.

Sample Plans and Introduction Scripts

Eduardo's Parents' Plan

- Week 1: Computer and gaming system will be removed from Eduardo's room. Computer will be set up in a common area of the house and password protected so that it can be used only for schoolwork. Eduardo can earn full use of the computer and use of the gaming system (also in a common area) when he attends a full day of school every day for 1 week (and continues to attend).

- Week 2: Mother will no longer take food to Eduardo's room.

- Week 3: Mother will no longer shower before entering Eduardo's room and will no longer do his laundry, make his bed, or clean his room.

- Week 4: Family no longer washes hands or uses hand sanitizer (unless after the bathroom, before meals, or if there's an actual illness going around).

- Week 5: No cleaning or washing places or items specially for Eduardo.

- Week 6: Anyone is welcome to visit our house and sit, touch, or go anywhere as long as it does not violate anyone else's privacy.

- Week 7: Toilets will be cleaned once a week (per the usual routine) instead of every day.

- Week 8: Mother pursues work outside the home.

At the beginning of week 1, Eduardo's mother and father approached Eduardo when he was in a calm mood and provided the following notification:

"Eduardo, a few days ago we let you know that we were going to be thinking about how we can help you get better at managing OCD. We know that your obsessions make you very anxious—they're the reason you've been staying in your room and missing school the last few months. But even though it seems like school and the rest of the house are contaminated, we know that you'd be OK if you left your room and spent time in these places. That's why, as a first step, we are taking away your computer and gaming system. The computer will be set up in the living room, and you will be able to use it only under supervision and for schoolwork. After you go back to school every day for a week, we will set up your gaming system in the living room and you'll be able to use it, and the computer, as much as you want as long as you're going to school every day. We understand this will be an adjustment, and we want you to know that we are not doing this to upset you. We love you very much and want to help you get back to school and get better. We would love for you to earn these things back as soon as possible." [Eduardo's parents had prearranged for two neighbors to help remove the computer and gaming system from Eduardo's room while he was taking a shower.]

Ariel's Husband's Plan

- Week 1: Stop providing reassurance that the doors are locked and everything is off.

- Week 2: Stop keeping a written log of Ariel's checking.

- Week 3: Stop going around the house with Ariel to check.

- Week 4: Stop leaving work to check for Ariel in the middle of the day.

- Week 5: Leave the house before Ariel in the morning if necessary.

- Week 6: Stop answering Ariel's calls or texts at work.

- Week 7. No more making excuses for Ariel if she's late for work.

One evening while Ben and Ariel were having dinner together (without their children present), Ben explained this plan to his wife:

"Ariel, I've had some time to think since we last talked about OCD, and I want to share my thoughts with you. You chose to marry me because of the values that we share. So I understand that you want me to help reassure you that everything is checked and safe at night—*even after you've checked everything.* But as you know, giving you reassurance isn't helping. That's why, as a first step, I've decided that I'm going to stop discussing these things with you before going to bed. Instead, it would be great if we could watch a show or talk about something else. If I ignore your reassurance-seeking questions or get up and walk away, it's not because I'm angry with you. It's because I love you too much to let this problem go on without doing something about it."

Xavier's Parents' Plan

- Week 1: Change to a church that is more in line with our religious views.

- Week 2: Keep Xavier on the payroll at the store only if he shows up for work every day. If he misses a day because of OCD, he is off the payroll.

- Week 3: Do not discuss or provide reassurance about God, sin, or faith, nor listen to confessions. Instead, answer questions by acknowledging Xavier's anxiety and uncertainty and his ability to manage this on his own.

- Week 4: Plan a vacation without Xavier.

Xavier's parents presented the following message to him when they were ready to begin implementing their plan:

"Xavier, I'm sure you remember our discussion about OCD last week. Since then, your mother and I have talked a lot about moving forward. As a first step, we have decided to attend a church that is more in line with our own preferences. We fully understand and respect if you want to remain at the church we've been attending—you are an adult, and that is your decision to make. But that church no longer works for Mother and me. We realize this might make you uncomfortable because we won't be able to analyze the pastor's sermons with you anymore. But we know how smart you are and trust that you will figure his messages out for yourself. That's why we are taking steps to help you become more independent. We will always love you very much."

Linda's Husband's Plan

- Week 1: Respond to reassurance seeking by only acknowledging Linda's fear and her ability to withstand anxiety.

- Week 2: Begin watching any TV shows I want to see; hang up pictures of Emma in the house; no more avoiding words or topics that provoke obsessional thoughts.

- Week 3: Refuse to make excuses for Linda if she is invited to see Emma.
- Week 4: Invite Emma's family to come to the house for a visit.

Nicholas informed Linda of his first accommodation reduction goal one afternoon when the couple was taking a walk outside together:

"Linda, after our talk about the obsessional thoughts the other day, I've been doing a lot of thinking. I know that these thoughts make you feel anxious and worried that you're a terrible person. And I know it feels like you need my reassurance. But my reassuring you only gives you temporary relief, and I know how strong you are and that you can get through that anxiety on your own and see that these thoughts are just nonsense. So, beginning now, I've decided not to give you reassurance about OCD thoughts anymore. It would be great if you would stop asking me for reassurance, but if you do ask, I will not answer your questions anymore. I know this may cause you anxiety, but as your husband who loves you very much, it's my job to help you get stronger in the face of these thoughts and the anxiety. Think of how much happier our family will be once we nip this in the bud together!"

What If Your Relative Gets Anxious or Asks for Accommodation?

Adjusting to the changes you're making might not be easy for your relative. He's likely to show signs of anxiety when you stop accommodating. She might continue to ask for "help" with avoidance, rituals, and other OCD-related behaviors. While Chapter 13 contains strategies for dealing with significant pushback, here is some advice for how to manage less serious circumstances. First, remember what you learned about anxiety, obsessional thoughts, and uncertainty back in Chapter 6: They're safe, temporary, and manageable. By ending accommodation, you're helping your loved one learn this, too. Next, draw on the communication skills you learned in Chapter 7 to respond in a supportive and assertive way. If he becomes anxious when you refuse to accommodate, remind him that you're confident he'll rally and get through the situation. If she continues to ask for accommodation, gently remind her that you've changed how you respond to such requests. It's about encouraging your relative to get through the distress rather than getting rid of the distress. Here are some examples:

- "I know how strong you are. You can do this—you can manage the anxiety!"

- "If I did that for you, it would only make the OCD stronger. Think of how proud you'll feel later on when you see that you can get through this without my help."

- "Remember that anxiety is safe and manageable. I know it feels uncomfortable, but I know you can handle it!"

- "We love you and we know this is difficult right now, but we've decided not to do these rituals anymore. You're strong and we know you can get through this."

- "It sounds like you're asking for reassurance, but I can't answer that for you. How can I help you without doing rituals for you?"

Evaluating Your Progress

After several weeks of working on reducing their accommodation, Xavier's parents were feeling discouraged. Xavier was still going to the same church, obsessing about whether he'd committed sins, and refusing to get treatment for OCD. Had anything changed? I reminded Xavier's parents that the goals they'd set were to change *their own* behavior—not Xavier's. And indeed, they'd been consistent in enacting their plan. Therefore, it was a mistake to base their judgment of progress on their son's behavior. Similarly, even if your family member doesn't respond the way you would like, you're making progress by simply sticking to your decision to change your own behavior. With this in mind, I recommend that at the end of each week you evaluate your progress based on the following questions:

- Where did you have the greatest success with reducing accommodation?

- Where did you come up short?

- What were the easiest and most difficult parts of changing your response to OCD?

- Were you able to be consistent with your behavior changes?

- Did you feel less involved in OCD than you have in the past?
- What strategies worked well and should be continued?
- What might you do differently in the upcoming week?

Really thinking through your answers to these questions will help you make adjustments and be even more successful in the weeks to come. And don't fall into the trap of minimizing small successes and magnifying disappointments! Stay focused on what went well and remind yourself that even the small triumphs add up and give you confidence.

Upon examining their situation more carefully, Xavier's parents actually had lots to be hopeful about. The fact that Xavier was attending a different church than his parents was a sign that he was becoming more independent. Furthermore, even though his obsessions persisted, his parents hadn't answered a reassurance-seeking question in weeks. They'd even planned a trip to visit family members for a few days without Xavier. Their son had clearly gained confidence in his ability to manage with anxiety, even if he was not yet ready to seek professional help. I encouraged Xavier's parents to catch Xavier in moments of success and give him lots of praise for his hard work, for example by saying things like:

- "We're very proud of you. We knew you could do it!"
- "Great job. I know this is not easy for you."
- "I really love how hard you're working on this."
- "I'm so happy that you chose to lean into the anxiety instead of asking for reassurance."

But getting to this point wasn't always smooth sailing for Xavier's parents, and most likely you'll also encounter some degree of pushback from your family member when you begin reducing accommodation. In the next chapter, I'll show you how to manage resistance and arguments, as well as more serious forms of escalation such as threats, violence, and other forms of extreme and inappropriate behavior.

12

Responding to Arguments, Threats, and Extreme Behavior

You probably don't need me to tell you that once you begin reducing accommodation, your loved one with OCD is likely to push back in one way or another. To her, obsessional fears are a danger signal, and your accommodation has been part of her safety net, so removing this net is not necessarily an easy adjustment for her. At the very least, you'll likely encounter verbal protests and arguments. Perhaps your son or daughter will turn to disruptive or aggressive behavior, or even threats of violence. A partner or spouse with OCD, however, is more likely to use emotional means to push back.

In this chapter, I'll first help you understand the psychology behind your loved one's pushback. Then I'll prepare you to respond to emotional pleas, arguments, disruptive behavior, and threats—including threats of self-harm and suicide—in ways that allow you to keep the situation from escalating while also accomplishing your goals of reducing accommodation and supporting your family member.

Understanding Pushback

Think of a vending machine you rely on regularly to deliver you a snack or a drink. Over and over again you feed it your money, push the button, and then out pops your snack. But then one day when you insert your money and hit the button, nothing comes out. What do you do? Maybe you push the button again and again. Still nothing? Maybe you pound on the machine with your fist. And if that doesn't work, you might try giving it an angry kick or two.

This is a classic example of what psychologists call an "extinction burst."

Extinction happens when you stop receiving something that you've come to expect—like the snack you've just paid for. The *burst* is your intensified effort to try to get it back. Because you've learned from experience that putting money in a vending machine results in receiving your food selection, you expect this to be the outcome every time. So when it doesn't happen, your behavior escalates (the "burst" of angry pushing and kicking) as you try to get the expected reward.

Do you see how this relates to OCD and accommodation? Perhaps your loved one has come to expect you or others to help control her anxiety or protect her from what she's afraid of. In other words, she *expects* to be accommodated. So when you begin withholding accommodation, she's likely to push back and protest in an extinction burst of her own. Yelling, arguing, name-calling, trying to make you feel guilty, throwing tantrums—they're all efforts to get you to go back to accommodating so that she can feel safe again.

Sometimes pushback involves more extreme behavior, such as making serious threats or committing actual physical aggression toward oneself, others, or property. These are most common among children, teens, and younger adults and less likely from a partner with OCD. Chances are you already have a good idea of how your loved one is likely to respond when you withhold accommodation.

As I've mentioned, it's important to keep in mind that pushback generally results from your relative's feelings of anxiety and fear, *not* from hatred or disrespect. In his mind, danger is present, so he's just doing what he believes is crucial to minimize his anxiety and the risk of harm to himself or others. In most cases, even more forceful and alarming responses are attempts to get you to give in and reduce his fear. Sure, your family member might say or do extremely disrespectful things during extinction bursts. But it's important not to take this too personally. Instead, consider the situation from *his* point of view: You've changed the rules and are now refusing to give him the one thing he's relied on to help him feel safe and comfortable. And just as you'll resort to banging and kicking that vending machine to try to get your snack, it's only natural that he'll try whatever he can—from self-pity to begging to intimidation—to get that accommodation back.

Fortunately, extinction bursts tend to be temporary—as long as you *don't* reward them by returning to accommodation or by taking them personally and overreacting to them. Give in, and you've taught your loved one that pushing back hard enough will eventually get you to abandon your plan and accommodate. Become angry or emotional, and he'll keep up the unpleasantness in hopes that you'll eventually throw in the towel. On the other hand, remaining calm and determined to teach your loved one that she can manage anxiety without accommodation will show her that pushback won't work. Eventually she'll give up—just as you'll ultimately walk away from the vending machine when your kicking and shoving prove ineffective. I'm not saying it's easy to resist pushback and extinction bursts (*you* have feelings . . . vending machines don't!), but it's critical for success and *you can do it*! So let's turn to different forms of pushback and the best ways to manage them.

Verbal Protests and Arguments

Tantrums

Remember Hannah, the 11-year-old with obsessional fears of odd numbers? She was assigned jersey #7 to wear on her soccer team. When her parents refused to ask the coach for an even-numbered jersey, Hannah began arguing that wearing jersey #7 would cause someone in their family to break their neck. Her parents' first instinct was to try to convince their daughter that her fear was senseless. But they wisely refused to get drawn into a debate about OCD and instead calmly explained that they understood she was anxious but were not going to allow her to change jerseys. That's when Hannah began screaming and crying—a full-blown extinction burst right there in front of her soccer team! She yelled at her parents, "You two are horrible people!" But her parents refused to make a big deal out of Hannah's spectacle. Instead, they quietly said, "We're going home. Are you coming with us?" and began walking toward the family car, talking to each other and ignoring Hannah's outburst. Hannah followed them, and after about 5 minutes of crying (which seemed more like 20 minutes!), she calmed down because she realized her parents were not going to give in. On the ride home there was no mention of Hannah's ugly display because her parents didn't want to reward this behavior by giving it any attention.

Like Hannah, your child with OCD might argue, protest, cry, or use tantrums to get you to give in and accommodate. If she knows you don't like it when she gets too anxious, she's likely to tell you how anxious she is. If she knows you don't like her saying that you don't love her, she'll tell you this as well. And if she thinks you'll respond to being cursed at and called names, she'll try that, too. As a rule, kids are smarter than we often give them credit for being, so be prepared and know what to expect so you're able to respond effectively. What's the most effective response?

Don't take the bait! Instead, ignore the pushback just as Hannah's parents did. Stay strong (grit your teeth if you have to) and don't take it personally.

Your job is to create a learning experience for your relative—a chance for her to see for herself that she doesn't need accommodation. Try to think of the extinction burst as your child's way of adapting to your new (and healthier) ways of responding to OCD. It's fine to distance yourself from your child by going into another room, going outside, or getting involved with some other person or activity. If she continues to argue, scream, or cry, that's OK. Your first instinct might be to yell at her or try to calm her down and give her the accommodation she wants to stop screaming. But remember that you don't have to do any of these things because your child's strong emotions will not harm her. What's more, yelling back or trying to calm her down are rewards in her eyes—she's getting your attention. If pushback is rewarded with any sort of reaction on your part, your family member will think she's got a chance to weaken your resolve, and she'll be encouraged to use the same approach next time. Yes, outbursts might have to get worse before they can get better, but they'll eventually stop when your child realizes she's not going to get your attention or your concession, so hang in there and be patient.

Get everyone on board. It might not be enough for just you to stop rewarding pushback. Instead, everyone in the family circle needs to follow the same approach for it to be successful. If one person gives in, your child will continue with his behavior, and extinction bursts will persist longer than they have to.

Passive–Aggressive Behavior

The pushback of an older son or daughter with OCD, perhaps an adult (child or partner), might look similar to that of a younger child but might also take a more discreet or sophisticated form. Passive–aggressive behavior demonstrates negative feelings but only in an indirect way. When Xavier's parents switched churches, Xavier pushed back using passive–aggressive comments that were intended to provoke his parents into a debate about religious observance and ultimately get them to come back to his church. For example, he'd say, "So much for 'a family that prays together stays together,' huh?" and "What kind of nonsense did your pastor brainwash you with today?" He'd also use two fingers of each hand to make quotation marks in the air ("air quotes") whenever he referred to his parents' church, as if to indicate that the word *church* didn't really apply to where they worshipped. When his parents failed to become agitated by these comments and gestures, Xavier escalated things by telling his parents they wouldn't be saved as Christians if they continued to attend their new church. This, he thought, would surely provoke a reaction. But Xavier's parents never relented. Even if they were bothered by Xavier's behavior, they never argued back or let on in any way that they were upset.

The next week, when Xavier was informed that he had to attend work to continue to receive a salary, he tried arguing with his mother on several occasions, listing all the reasons that this change was unfair. A few times Xavier burst into tears and raised his voice. Even though this was extremely difficult for her to witness, Xavier's mother responded like a broken record every time, calmly stating, "We love you, Xavier. And your father and I are determined to help you become more independent." Then she smiled and walked away, leaving Xavier to himself. Within a few days, the arguing and tears had stopped, and Xavier began showing up for work.

Tugging at Your Emotions

Similar to passive–aggressive behavior, it's possible that your loved one— particularly an older child, partner, or spouse—will use emotional strategies to try to get you to change your behavior and resume accommodation. He might plead with you, "If you really loved me, you would do this for me," or say things like "You don't care about me." When this happens, it's important to keep in mind that he's using these strategies because he thinks they'll get you to change your behavior (maybe it's worked in the past). But just as you read about in Chapter 10 on establishing and maintaining boundaries, it's important not to take these responses personally. That is, don't fall into the trap of arguing or trying to reassure your child or partner that you *do* love him. This kind of attention and will only teach him that tugging at your emotions will work; so he'll do it again and again. Instead, try to see his actions for what they really are—a response to anxiety and fear. Then, calmly let him how that you understand he's feeling anxious, remind him that you're no longer accommodating his OCD symptoms, explain why you've decided to stop accommodating, and suggest an alternative activity that you both might enjoy.

At one point, Linda became anxious about having pictures of Emma on the wall and accused Nicholas of not being a loving husband: "You know how anxious these pictures make me. If you really loved me, you wouldn't put them up on the wall." But rather than reassuring her, or taking down the pictures, Nicholas said, "Linda, I know pictures of Emma make you anxious, but I've decided that I'm no longer going to help you avoid these pictures because avoidance only makes your OCD worse. Maybe you'd feel better if we take a walk or do some yardwork together. Will you join me?" If Linda continued to tug at Nicholas's emotions, he used the broken record technique from

Chapter 7 so that Linda eventually learned that using this strategy wouldn't get her husband to go back to accommodating.

Debates about Risk and Safety

Another common mistake is to engage in debates about risk and safety with your family member. When Eduardo argued that bathrooms are unsafe and that the germs found there would make him very sick, it was difficult for his father to resist using logic to convince his son that he'd be just fine. They'd go back and forth, his father arguing that people generally don't get sick from using the bathroom and Eduardo coming up with reasons to discount what his father was saying. As you've read, OCD doesn't respond to logic, so it's no use arguing about risk with your family member. Not only that, when you debate with your loved one, you send the message that you're not completely certain of your decision to stop accommodating. This weakens your position.

So what *is* the best way to respond when your loved one pushes back by arguing that reducing accommodation could cause something awful to happen? Remember that uncertainty is ubiquitous and that you're helping your relative get better at managing acceptable levels of uncertainty and risk. So there's no need to try to convince her that everything is going to be OK (after all, you don't have a guarantee either!). Therefore, defuse the argument by agreeing with her that there *is* some risk. Here are some examples:

- "You're right, bathroom germs *could* make you sick. And I get that you're genuinely afraid of them. As your parent, it's my job to help you get better at managing this kind of everyday risk."

- "You've got a point. There's no such thing as 100% safe. There's *some* risk to just about everything, and I understand this situation makes you feel very anxious. And just like in other situations, I know you can handle the uncertainty here too."

- "I'm not going to argue with you about risk because we've been down that road. But I know the risk is reasonably low and you can manage this."

The Silent Treatment

When Ben stopped responding to Ariel's reassurance-seeking texts and phone calls during the work day, Ariel pushed back by giving Ben the cold shoulder. She ignored his questions and comments, rejected any sort of physical or emotional affection, refused to speak to him at the dinner table, walked away if he entered the room she was in, and even began sleeping in a different room. The only time Ariel briskly communicated with Ben was when it regarded their children. This went on for a few days.

Your partner with OCD might resort to some of the types of pushback already described. But, like Ariel, she might also give you the silent treatment when you stop accommodating her anxiety. Some older children might use this strategy as well. This silent treatment (or what psychologists call *withholding*) is your loved one's attempt to regain control of a situation in which she feels scared, vulnerable, or hurt. In a way, this is understandable coming from someone whose protection from obsessional fear has been taken away. But the silent treatment is an unhealthy communication pattern.

If your *child* is giving you the silent treatment, my advice is not to do anything at all except continue working toward your accommodation reduction goals. Don't take it personally—instead, try to see his withholding behavior as a sign that he has the ability to be independent. Sooner or later he'll most likely need to communicate with you, and you should reengage with him as if nothing has happened, without even mentioning the silent treatment he's been giving you.

On the other hand, if the silent treatment is coming from your *partner*, it's worth addressing directly. Poor communication patterns can develop into habits that have longer-term impacts on your relationship (and your children, if you have them). Fortunately, the cold shoulder is not difficult to deal with. Here's how:

- **Label your experiences.** Open the door to healthy communication by acknowledging how you're feeling. Keep it simple and avoid accusations or hostile language. For example, "Hey, I noticed you're not responding to me." But don't push the issue. If he doesn't respond immediately, give him some time and try again later.

- **Listen assertively.** Use the assertive listening skills on pages 95–97 in Chapter 7 to validate her experiences and create space for conversation.

- **Share your thoughts and feelings.** For example, say something like "I know when I stop talking to someone it means that I'm feeling angry, upset, or sad. If you need space and you're not ready to talk, I understand. But the silence is hard for me. Maybe we can find a time to talk about this." When the time comes, make sure to assertively explain your position regarding OCD and accommodation using "*I* statements."

- **Avoid future silent treatment.** Routinely tell your loved one what you're thinking and feeling using the communication skills you learned in Chapter 7. Hopefully this will help your partner do the same in return.

Unruly or Violent Behavior

Eduardo would become infuriated and act out when his mother refused to bring food to his room. The violent screaming and cursing would go on and on. Sometimes, he would aggressively slam doors, knock over furniture, and throw books and other objects around the house. These tantrums sometimes resulted in serious damage. Eduardo was also taller than both his mother and his sister, and would sometimes lunge and grab at them as if to intimidate them with his size. He began making angry threats toward his sister when she refused to give in to Eduardo's demand that she wash her hands. For example, he'd say things like "If I were you, I'd sleep with one eye open tonight." Eduardo's parents were extremely concerned and had second thoughts about the safety of continuing with their accommodation reduction plan. Had they made their situation worse? How would they continue with their plan knowing it could trigger Eduardo to engage in violence?

Aggressive behavior is a common response to anxiety—it's the "fight" part of the fight-or-flight response. When your relative is less anxious, he'll become less unruly. But it's important to let this process play out naturally, rather than trying to directly calm your loved one down while he's acting out as this will only increase his aggression. In the heat of the moment it's difficult for your child to maintain self-control, plus he'll misperceive anything you say as a challenge (even something as passive as "Let's all settle down"), which will further escalate his anger. And since *you're* probably wound up as well, it's likely you'll respond in exaggerated ways, further fueling the situation. Instead, here's what to do.

Get Some Physical Distance

The fact is, since you can't directly control your child's behavior, there's really no good way to respond in the moment to stop unruliness. Of course, you'll respond later—once she has had a chance to calm down. But in the moment, you've simply got to focus on not getting pulled into the conflict. Your best option, therefore, is to physically distance yourself from your child. If she makes threats, try to stay silent (or calmly remind him that the behavior is unacceptable). Whatever you do, avoid making threats in return (such as "You'll be sorry if you _____!") as this will only feed her aggression. Your goal is to allow the natural calming process to take its course. Although it might seem counterintuitive not to intervene at this point, it's the best way to foster your child's coping and self-regulation skills.

Of course, you also have the right to feel physically safe. So if your family member becomes violent toward you or anyone else, seek help; call an advocate, or even the police (dial 911), if necessary. It doesn't mean that you don't love your child; the safety of you and your family should always come first.

Hold a Sit-In

Psychologists Eli Lebowitz and Haim Omer recommend waiting for at least a few hours after an episode of severe unruly or violent behavior and then holding a "sit-in" to let your son or daughter know that such behavior is not acceptable. The benefit of this strategy is that it shows you're committed to eliminating the behavior without escalating the conflict. Here are the steps they suggest:

- Prepare to spend up to an hour with your child, which means you might need to arrange for child care if there are other children in your home. If you have a co-parent, he or she should accompany you at the sit-in.

- Enter your loved one's room and sit down. Make sure neither you nor your child is feeling angry at this point.

- In a calm tone, explain that you're there because of her violent behavior and you're determined to solve the problem. For example, say something like "Yesterday, when Mother refused to do your laundry a second time, you opened the container of detergent and threw it at her. This is unacceptable, and we will stay here and wait for you to suggest a solution to this problem. We are not punishing you, but we cannot accept this kind of behavior in our home."

- Remain in your child's room quietly for up to 1 hour (you can reduce this to a half hour if your child is younger than 12) and do not respond to any provocation or demands that you leave the room.

- If your child makes what seems like a reasonable suggestion for how she'll manage the next time there's a conflict over OCD and accommodation, say that you agree to try that solution next time and then leave the room quietly. Don't discuss the sit-in after it's over, even if your child threatens to rescind the solution she proposed.

- Repeat the sit-in only if the child acts violently again; but this time do not leave until a completely new solution has been proposed.

You might also involve your advocates in the sit-in, or at least notify them of the violent behavior. Informing your child that the outside individual knows the details of his unacceptable behavior can be a strong deterrent of future violence. For example, you might say something like "We will not keep it a secret when you act this way. Therefore, we have let Uncle Roy know about what happened." You can also encourage the advocate to contact your child directly to express care and concern, offer to help, and show support for how you're managing the situation.

Threats of Suicide or Self-Harm

"I'll kill myself if you don't help with my rituals."

Hearing a family member threaten self-harm or suicide seems like a no-win situation. You're worried about what he'll do, and you feel responsible for having caused him to feel this way. But if you back down and do whatever seems necessary to reduce his distress, you'll teach him that making these kinds of threats (whether or not they're legitimate) is a good way to coax you into accommodating his OCD. And if it works once or twice, he's likely to play this card again and again. On the other hand, maybe you've considered calling his bluff and saying something like "The knives are in the kitchen. Go help yourself!" But what if he isn't bluffing? Are you really qualified to make that determination? Without a professional's opinion, it's never a good idea to ignore threats of self-harm. So mocking or daring your loved one isn't a good solution.

Katie avoided handling food because of obsessional fears that she would inadvertently poison herself and her family. Her husband, Steve, had taken on all of the responsibilities around meal preparation at home, including extensive washing and checking under Katie's close supervision. When Steve began cutting back on this accommodation, Katie threatened to stop eating because of her extreme fear of becoming ill. Steve was determined, but after more than a week of refusing to eat, Katie began to appear weak and undernourished. Steve became worried. Maybe stopping the accommodation was the wrong thing to do. Maybe he was making the problem worse and should give in to Katie's OCD so she'd begin eating again.

Keep in mind that in addition to helping your loved one learn healthy ways of managing obsessional fear and imagined threats, it's also your role as a parent or a partner to protect her from *real* threats—including herself. Therefore, the supportive response to threats of self-harm or suicide is to remain determined not to accommodate OCD *while at the same time taking her threats seriously.* In other words, just as you wouldn't give in and help with rituals when your relative says she's "very anxious," you can also refuse to accommodate when she's threatening self-harm—the difference being that you must also make sure to keep her safe.

Seeking Emergency Services

Bearing all of this in mind, your best bet is to seek emergency medical attention for your loved one if he makes threats of self-harm. This is true regardless of whether he's a child or an adult. Once a threat is made, begin by *calmly* explaining that you take his safety very seriously and because you're so concerned, you must do whatever you can to prevent tragedy. In most cases, this means taking the person to the nearest emergency room, where a mental health crisis professional will conduct a risk assessment. When Steve became concerned about Katie's weight loss, he took her to an emergency room. Her blood was drawn and she was thoroughly evaluated, including by a psychiatrist. Although the blood tests came back normal, they indicated borderline low levels of some important nutrients; and when Katie heard that the doctors were thinking of admitting her to the hospital for a few days, she immediately promised to start eating normally—which is exactly what she did.

If going to the emergency room is not possible, calling 911, explaining to the switchboard operator that your loved one is threatening self-harm or suicide, and asking for a paramedic with crisis intervention training to come to your residence is an appropriate alternative. Keep your composure throughout the process. This is not a punishment for your family member—you are taking action in response to an emergency.

I realize that calling 911 or going to an emergency room might seem dramatic, but there are several reasons it's worth the time and energy to have your loved one evaluated by a professional. First, it frees *you* from having to guess how serious she is about harming herself—which you're most likely not qualified to determine on your own. What's more, if your relative really is a danger to herself, the hospital is the safest place for her to be. If, on the other hand, the risk is determined by a professional to be low, you can confidently return to your accommodation reduction plan knowing that your loved one has been evaluated properly. Finally, because the hospital visit is not a response that rewards threats of self-harm, your family member will be less likely to use these threats in the future. Katie, for example, realized that refusing to eat would land her in the hospital—where she didn't want to be. And on the way home, Steve reminded her that he'd always take threats of harm seriously. You should do the same with your relative and make sure never to threaten to use emergency room visits as a punishment. This will ruin the effects of the visit and leave you with few options to deal with future threats.

There's a good chance your relative will try to take back his threat when you tell him you're taking him to the emergency room. He might even try to call *your* bluff by agreeing to go to the hospital right up until he realizes you're serious about taking him. At first, Katie pleaded with Steve to reconsider and even swore that she'd start eating again. But once you've let your family member know of your intention, it's important to follow through regardless of how much she tries to recant. You might say, for example, "Maybe you didn't mean to say that you were thinking of suicide, but I love you too much to just ignore something like that." Steve told Katie, "You're too important to me. I can't let you starve yourself." Your relative will learn that suicidal threats (and other self-injurious behaviors) are too serious to be "taken back," which will encourage him to think twice about them in the future.

Responding to Emotional Blackmail

If your loved one with OCD is an adult who regularly threatens self-harm whenever you're doing something she doesn't like (especially after a trained professional has determined that she is at low risk for hurting herself), she's likely trying to take advantage of your love and concerns about her safety. This is emotional blackmail—a form of abuse—and here's how to handle it:

- **Stick to your boundaries.** Giving in to these kinds of threats over and over only makes you angry and resentful. Instead, say something like "I care about you very much, and I understand you're upset right now, but I will not help you do rituals."

- **You don't have to prove your love.** You don't owe your loved one "proof" that you love her when she says things like "If you really loved me, you'd stop me from killing myself" (ironically, it's *she* who is not showing *you* love). Instead, put the choice back on her. It's OK to respond by saying something like "I really care about you, but this is your choice, and I can't stop you from making it."

- **Focus on your own well-being.** Whether it's a serious threat or a recurring bluff, hearing a loved one speak of suicide can be an enormous source of stress. So in addition to the tips I've suggested in this chapter, review the material in Chapter 5 on taking care of yourself and managing stress. Finally, consider talking with a professional therapist if you feel like the stress is getting the better of you.

I hope you won't have to deal with pushback and extinction bursts, nor use the strategies I've described in this chapter for too long before your relative with OCD catches on and begins cooperating with you. When you establish new responses to pushback, and remain consistent in how you handle extinction bursts, she'll learn what to expect from you and begin to problem-solve on her own. Sure, there will be bumps in the road—just about every family I've worked with has them. But once things begin moving in the right direction, you can use the strategies in the next chapter to keep your program on track.

13

Staying on Track

As you've become less involved in your loved one's OCD symptoms, I hope you've also noticed an increase in your self-confidence. Your family or relationship environment has likely improved as well, and you may feel better about tending to your own needs and less worried about your loved one with OCD. And although you've been focused on changing your own approach, I hope this program has also translated to changes in your relative's ability to manage OCD symptoms more independently.

But this is an ongoing process, and as you set and work toward more goals you'll also need to focus on maintaining the changes you've made. In this chapter, I'll help you stay on track by taking stock of how far you've come and where you've made less progress. You'll also reward your loved one for showing confidence and independence, inject productive ways to fill the gaps left by OCD, and stay alert for lapses and setbacks while preventing full-blown relapses.

Assessing Your Progress

As I mentioned in Chapter 11, one strategy to help you stay on track is to periodically assess your progress. So, at the end of every week, take some time to reflect on the changes you've been making and their impact. I recommend starting with a review of the accommodation reduction goals you set back on page 149. Which goals have you been working toward, and how much headway have you made in achieving them? You can use the form on page 183 to rate your progress with each goal from 0 (no progress) to 8 (goal achieved). You might want to make copies of this form so you can use it periodically.

In assessing your progress, it can be helpful to ask yourself the following questions:

What effects have the changes you've been making had on your ability to support your loved one? How much more confident have you become responding to her anxiety without feeling like you need to immediately reduce her distress? If you're a parent, how much do you feel that you've been able to assume a healthier role as a mother or father? What about as a partner or spouse of someone with OCD? How have your feelings about your relative changed? Do you think of her as more capable of coping with anxiety? Are you able to disengage from OCD when you wish to and enjoy things that are important to you?

How have the changes you've been making impacted your loved one? Has he become more tolerant of anxiety, obsessional thoughts, or uncertainty? Has he become more independent and better able to regulate his responses to distressing situations, thoughts, and feelings? Maybe he's doing fewer rituals and avoiding fewer situations. How much has his general self-confidence and self-esteem improved? How about improvement in other areas of his functioning? Does he see himself as making progress and feeling better? It's also important to think about where things haven't improved and what work still needs to be done. By working toward your goals, you're helping your family member with OCD develop skills that he'll use for a lifetime.

How have your changes impacted life in your household more generally? Are things more peaceful? Are people getting along better? Is there more cooperation? Are you able to be on time for important commitments? You might flip back to the Impact of OCD Rating Form you filled out in Chapter 8 (pages 103–104) and complete this form again to give you an idea of how much your hard work is paying off when it comes to your family or relationship. Where do you notice the most change? Where are difficulties still cropping up? Keeping up with these ratings can also help you make decisions about what to target next.

Rewarding Yourself

Be sure to reward yourself for reducing accommodation and stimulating changes in your household—not only because it will make you feel good but also because it will motivate you to work even harder. Make your rewards meaningful and enjoyable and match the size of the rewards to the size of the goals reached. Here are some examples.

Working toward Accommodation Reduction Goals

Rate how much progress you've made toward achieving your goals for reducing accommodation using the scale below.

0	1	2	3	4	5	6	7	8
No progress		A little progress		Moderate progress		A great deal of progress		Goal achieved!

Accommodation reduction goal	Rating

- Buy something for your hobby
- Enjoy a nice meal at a fancy restaurant
- See a movie
- Go for a spa treatment or massage
- Attend a show or concert you've been wanting to see
- Pay someone to do the yardwork or housecleaning this week
- Find some time to be by yourself
- Take a weekend getaway

What If You're Not Where You Want to Be?

Reducing accommodation is no small task, so your progress might be slower than you had hoped. But don't beat yourself up about the challenges you haven't overcome yet. Keep up your efforts and try to pinpoint obstacles and other challenges that might have limited your success in implementing and sticking with your plan:

- Maybe you didn't realize how upset or anxious your loved one would become and you began to second-guess yourself and your plan.
- Maybe your relative threatened you or said something to make you feel guilty.
- Maybe you personalized something she said and got drawn into an argument.
- Maybe you put pressure on yourself to move too quickly and try to make too many changes at once.

Once you've identified possible barriers to your success, consider these possibilities for dismantling them:

- Go back to earlier chapters in this book to review the facts about OCD, anxiety, and effective communication strategies.
- If a particularly threatening or aggressive response from your relative has hampered progress, review the strategies in Chapter 12 for dealing with these types of responses.

- Could an advocate (described in Chapter 9) help with aggression from your relative?

- It's never a bad idea to seek professional help from an experienced family or couple therapist who specializes in CBT for OCD and anxiety and will know how to work with you on the particular problem you're dealing with. Chapter 14 can help you locate an appropriate professional.

Whatever solution you choose, revise your plan and then try implementing it once again. Repeat this process until you're satisfied and ready to move on to your next goal.

What If Your Family Member Isn't Where You Want Him to Be?

Maybe you've achieved all of your goals and successfully disentangled yourself from OCD, but your relative hasn't responded the way you'd like. Perhaps he's still avoiding obsessional triggers and doing compulsive rituals, but without involving you or other family members. Maybe he continues to turn down opportunities to get professional help. It's also possible he's become increasingly withdrawn, indifferent to rewards and consequences, and seemingly content to live with OCD. He might blame others for his problems, refuse to work or go to school, and expect you to take responsibility for him. Experts sometimes refer to this scenario as "failure to launch" because it most often occurs among young adults who have trouble starting a life of their own. Although your relative's OCD symptoms might not directly affect you the way they once did, you remain deeply troubled with how his problem interferes with his own functioning and threatens his chances of having a normal life.

Since you can't control your "adult" child, the most difficult part of this situation is accepting his unfortunate decision to live this way even if it's not what you want. Don't fall into the trap of blaming yourself—you're not responsible for your relative's choices; and in fact you've been working hard to support him. And don't let yourself think that you've got to suffer along with your relative. Just because he isn't willing to do something about his problem doesn't mean you have to stop living your life. Here are some ways you can use the advice in this book if you find yourself in this situation—and don't be afraid to seek professional help as well (perhaps with a partner):

- Make sure you're taking care of yourself both mentally and physically. Use the strategies in Chapter 5 to help you manage stress and feel better about living your own life.

- Extend your refusal to accommodate beyond OCD. Resist the urge to cook meals for your adult child, do her laundry, or keep track of any medical appointments. It might seem important to ensure she's healthy, fed, and groomed, but enabling her in these ways will only keep her from learning how to manage for herself.

- Decide what behavior you will and won't tolerate and set clear boundaries and expectations for what's required to live under your roof (Chapter 10). Some parents make the decision that their adult children are no longer welcome to live in their home.

- Don't protect him from making mistakes or from failing, which are normal parts of life. Instead, help him see letdowns as opportunities to learn and grow.

- Continue to find ways to use rewards to encourage healthy behavior, as described in the next section.

Rewarding Your Loved One's Progress

I've already stressed the importance of catching your loved one in the act of doing something good. This recommendation applies as strongly as ever now that there's less accommodation in your home. Although you can't directly change her behavior, rewards boost your loved one's confidence, improve your relationship, and encourage healthy responses to obsessions and anxiety until this behavior becomes part of who she is. When you give a reward, your relative knows that you've noticed her doing something you like. This leads to positive feelings—not only for your loved one, but also for yourself.

If you need a refresher on giving rewards, review pages 137–142. But now that's you're reducing accommodation, be on the lookout for these three types of behaviors that you'll want to reward:

- **Distress tolerance.** Try to catch your family member showing greater tolerance for anxiety, obsessional thoughts, and uncertainty by acting in nonanxious ways—or even *leaning into* anxiety—instead of trying to avoid or escape from it. For example, even though she feels very anxious and uncertain, Ariel resists the urge to ask Ben to help her check (or even to check at all).

- **Confidence and independence.** Reward behaviors that indicate your relative is becoming more self-reliant, independent, and self-confident in other ways. For example, she does chores around the house, goes to bed on her own, or does schoolwork independently. Xavier's parents rewarded their son when he started showing up for work consistently.

- **Managing with the new normal.** Look for times when your loved one shows that he's managing with the changes you've made. But don't require him to be *enthusiastic* about managing—any sign that he's *dealing with* your changes should be enough to earn a reward. Eduardo, for example, wasn't exactly thrilled when his mother stopped cleaning the bathroom for him every morning, but after a while he stopped arguing and coped with this reality. Any sign of cooperation, including fewer arguments or extinction bursts, is a good thing to reward.

Look for opportunities to give rewards; but make sure to be genuine. Eduardo's mother, for example, shouldn't exclaim, "You did a terrific job getting ready for school this morning!" if in fact Eduardo spent an hour yelling at her because she refused to clean the toilet for him. Instead, she might say, "I'm proud of you for using the bathroom even though I didn't clean it first— that must have been difficult for you." Notice that Eduardo's mother found a way to socially reward Eduardo for "handling" the refusal to accommodate even though he didn't handle it particularly well. As another example, Ben ended up sleeping on the couch one evening because Ariel was furious that he wouldn't help with her checking rituals. In the end, however, Ariel went to bed without checking. The next morning, when she approached Ben cautiously, he responded with a big hug. Ariel was puzzled: "I thought you would still be angry about last night." But Ben specifically pointed out that Ariel had made progress: "I didn't like all the nasty stuff you said, but in the end you went to bed without checking—and that's amazing! I know you can do this!"

Introducing "OCD–Incompatible" Behaviors to Fill the Void

As you reduce accommodation, the space that's left could easily be filled with other problematic behavior patterns. So now that Eduardo is able to leave his room, what activities can he get involved with (besides going to school)? And once Xavier is no longer spending hours discussing his fears about God with his parents, what will he do with this extra time? Left to their own devices, both of these people, and your relative, might come up with other OCD-based strategies to reduce their obsessional fear, such as calling other people and asking them for assurances or going online (for example, to OCD or religious discussion forums) to read about scrupulosity. Like Eduardo's and Xavier's parents, you'll want to help your family member replace OCD symptoms with behaviors that promote a healthier lifestyle—what I call "OCD-incompatible behaviors." For Eduardo, this might include joining a club at school. For Xavier, this might include exercising after work.

Along the same lines, if accommodating OCD has become an important way you express care and concern for your spouse or partner, cutting back may disrupt your sense of togetherness. Recall from Chapter 12, for example, that Ariel gave Ben the cold shoulder when he stopped accommodating. In such instances, it's important to think about new OCD-incompatible ways to express care and concern and feel close to each other. Ben and Ariel, for instance, had shared a large amount of their time at home doing checking rituals together. Ben came to see "helping" with rituals as a way of showing Ariel how much he loved her. He knew that cutting down on this accommodation was the right thing to do, but he also needed to find new, more supportive ways to show Ariel that he loved her.

Although you can't demand that your relative engage in OCD-incompatible behaviors, there are supportive ways to encourage healthier living and express your love. One way is to invite your family member to engage in meaningful joint activities with you. Sometimes changing up the usual routine is exactly what's needed to turn the page on old habits. Here are some examples of healthy activities you and your loved one (or your entire family) could engage in to fill the void left by OCD behaviors:

- Attend a concert
- Take a class
- Exercise or go to the gym
- Prepare a special meal together
- Play a game together
- Go to a movie or play
- Work on a scrapbook or photo album
- Work on home improvement projects or do yardwork together
- Learn or play musical instruments together
- Visit friends or relatives

- Engage in physical intimacy
- Go shopping
- Go for a walk or out for a drive
- Volunteer together in the community

Another supportive way to encourage healthy behavior is to show your relative that facing fears, unwanted thoughts, and uncertainties without overreacting is indeed achievable. Psychologists call this *modeling*. Nicholas showed Linda that he was willing to experience discomfort by suggesting that they join a fitness club together—something Linda had always wanted to do but Nicholas avoided because he was out of shape and a bit self-conscious. Of course, he didn't do this to rub it in his wife's face ("See, look what I can do!"), but rather to model an appropriate response to feeling self-conscious and unsure of himself. Another important benefit of modeling is that it's a show of solidarity against OCD. That is, by confronting your own discomfort, it's as if you're telling your loved one, "I know this isn't easy for you, so the least I can do is step out of my own comfort zone as well." To this end, look for opportunities to demonstrate for your relative the ability to tactfully manage anxiety and fear. Seek out situations in which you can model calm, accepting, and discreet responses to unpleasant thoughts, imperfection, dirtiness, doubt, uncertainty, and the like.

Finally, you can also use rewards to incentivize OCD-incompatible behavior. If you're the parent of a child with OCD, set up a system where your son or daughter earns something tangible (for example, stickers or money) for engaging in healthy non-OCD behavior instead of ritualizing. This will help him feel better about his decision to approach discomfort and uncertainty rather than trying to fight these experiences.

Managing Lapses and Preventing Relapses

Even with rewards, troubleshooting, and anti-OCD behaviors, it's normal to hit bumps in the road as you work toward your accommodation reduction goals. This section presents some strategies to help you manage these hurdles and keep things moving in the right direction.

Lapses and Relapses

Simply put, a lapse is a slip—a noticeable increase in accommodating OCD after you've started making real progress in reducing accommodation.

Nicholas had made great strides in reducing his accommodation of Linda's obsessional thoughts and fears regarding her granddaughter but realized one day that he had reassured Linda five times that she wasn't a sexual predator and would never hurt Emma. This was the first signal that Nicholas was experiencing a lapse.

Lapses are not by themselves cause for too much alarm. However, if they become frequent, and more the rule than the exception, you may be headed for a *relapse*—a much more serious return to the accommodation patterns of the past that are harder to control. Almost all relapses can be prevented. The important thing is to notice the early warning signs. Understanding what causes lapses and relapses is the first step to keeping them in check.

A number of factors can lead to lapses and relapses. Increased stress in your home is one of the big ones. Stressful events lower your resistance and sap your energy, leaving you more susceptible to unhelpful thinking and acting patterns, as well as to arguments and other forms of pushback from your family member with OCD. Incidents that coincide with this family member's obsessional fears can also trigger lapses. Nicholas's lapse occurred after he and Linda saw a story on the news about a local sexual predator who had been arrested. Eduardo's mother lapsed into accommodating her son's fears of contamination when he developed a minor eye infection. A lapse is understandable following coincidences like these. But it doesn't mean you're back to square one. Since you've tackled accommodation once, doing it again should be even easier.

Your loved one might also contribute to lapses by testing you from time to time. That is, because at times he still has obsessional thoughts and feels anxious, he may seize on opportunities to see if you'll return to helping with (or putting up with) avoidance, rituals, or other OCD-related behaviors that you had previously stopped accommodating. Your daughter who'd stopped demanding that family members wash their hands might try to get them to decontaminate for her once again. Your husband who'd seemingly ended his rituals of repeating everything three times might go back to doing them, often making you late.

How to Prevent Relapse

Relapse prevention starts with being proactive and remaining aware of those situations likely to cause stress or trigger a lapse. You should also remain on the lookout for warning signs and approach the lapse as a temporary setback that you know how to overcome. Then you can use the skills and strategies you learned throughout this book to turn things around. Here are the strategies I've found effective for identifying and dealing with lapses:

Identify high-risk situations. Since the chances of a lapse increase when there's more stress in your household, you don't have to get taken by surprise. Has there recently been a family health issue or crisis? Have you lost a close relative or had a close relationship come to an end? Have work, school, or financial pressures increased? These are examples of negative stressors, but positive events that require adjustments can also produce stress. Is someone starting a new job? Have you recently gotten married? Had a new baby? Any events or situations that require change for you or other members of your family are potential high-risk situations because they increase the odds of a lapse. When you know such an event is coming up, prepare yourself for a possible return to accommodation. If you're prepared, the lapse won't catch you off guard and you'll be ready to take action immediately. You might think about some stressful high-risk situations that you anticipate in the next few months.

Spot the warning signs. Before you can prevent a relapse, you need to identify the signs that a lapse is occurring. Here are some warning signs:

- Feeling afraid your loved one's anxiety or obsessions are becoming "too intense"
- Feeling like you have to oversee or supervise your loved one
- Constantly putting your loved one's needs ahead of yours
- Feeling more irritable or feeling down
- Noticing more stress in relationships among family members due to OCD
- Having family routines once again become affected by OCD

Stay positive. Don't fall into the trap of panicking or beating up on yourself. Remember that lapses are normal and unavoidable. They occur sometimes despite your best intentions. Saying things to yourself such as "Oh no, I'm failing!" or "This is awful; I can't take this again" will only lead you into a cycle of despair and increase your stress. And remember that stress increases the chances of returning to accommodating. Instead of heaping criticism on yourself, keep calm and take action. The following coping statements might help you deal effectively with a lapse:

- "Everything's OK. This was bound to happen. Everyone has lapses."

- "I'm glad I caught this before it got out of control. I know what I have to do now."

- "For whatever reason, I'm having some trouble with giving in. I guess it means I need to work a little harder."

- "I've been successful with this before. There's no reason I can't do it again!"

Take action. Don't allow your loved one to believe that you're OK with the old behavior patterns you've worked so hard to change. Even if it means she'll become upset, it's important that you let her know you're confident she can handle the anxiety. If you're firm and self-assured, the lapse will pass much more quickly than if you're worried about provoking discomfort. You might say, for example, "It looks like an obsession has come up. That's OK, but I know you can manage this." Then use the strategies I've outlined in the preceding chapters to get things back on track.

Make sure to assess your progress. Assessing your progress periodically is one of the best ways to protect against relapse. You should especially check up on how you're doing during or after a particularly stressful time in your home, since these events increase the risk of lapses.

• • •

You've now got the information and strategic knowledge to plan, implement, troubleshoot, and maintain a program for getting you and your family disentangled from OCD while providing the healthiest kind of support for your family member—the kind of support in which anxiety, obsessions, and uncertainty are considered safe and normal. The kind of program in which the goal is not necessarily to have a loved one who is obsession-free, but one who is better able to manage obsessions and therefore prepared for what's in store on the road of life ahead. As I've mentioned, you'll have successes and challenges along the way. But by focusing on changing only your own behavior you're likely to see improvement, first and foremost, in your confidence and ability to reduce accommodation and shrink your involvement in your loved one's OCD symptoms. This, in turn, should lead to improvements in the overall operation of your household and to feeling more comfortable living your life and taking care of your needs.

Although you can't directly control your family member, another effect of your hard work is that it increases her incentive to seek (or be receptive to) professional help. Here's what I mean: when she recognizes that getting others to accommodate her OCD symptoms is no longer an option, but that there's hope for learning how to manage these symptoms, become more independent, and improve her quality of life, the prospect of overcoming OCD will begin to look more favorable than the status quo. Of course, I can't guarantee this outcome, but it is where many families I've worked with end up. That's why I've included the chapters in Part IV of this book. They'll give you the information you need to coach and support your loved one should she decide to pursue formal treatment.

PART IV

When Your Loved One Is Ready for Help

14

Finding the Right Treatment Program and Provider

Your family member has made the decision to get professional help . . . terrific! So what's next? The first step is deciding on what level of treatment to pursue. Then you've got to locate a clinician. The task of finding treatment for OCD might seem as simple as getting a referral or searching online and then scheduling an appointment . . . but it's not. You might encounter "specialists" whose actual knowledge of OCD and its treatment falls short, clinicians who state that they know how to do ERP but don't have the proper training, or those who offer sensible-sounding treatments (or treatments that are appealing because they don't involve exposure to feared situations) but have no scientific evidence of effectiveness for OCD. Therefore, it's important to be able to make sense of what you see and hear on websites and in directories. The goal of this chapter is to make you an informed consumer so you can:

1. Make decisions about treatment intensity.

2. Locate and interview treatment providers to make sure your family member ends up working with a capable clinician.

3. Sift out experimental and unproven therapies and avoid spending lots of time, effort, and money for a "treatment" that's unlikely to benefit your loved one.

What's the Right Type of Program for Your Relative?

Should your relative see a therapist once each week? Multiple times per week? Would she be better off with residential treatment? Carefully conducted clinical trials have shown that CBT (specifically ERP) can be delivered effectively through different types of programs that range from extremely hands-off to highly supervised. Variations in intensity and other factors you should consider when thinking about which method is best for your relative are discussed below.

Self-Help

Many authors and experts (including me) have packaged the techniques of CBT (especially ERP) into books, smartphone applications, and online programs. The International OCD Foundation (IOCDF) maintains a database of these resources at *https://iocdf.org/help*). The advantages of a self-help approach include that it's less costly, more efficient, and more accessible than working with a therapist (depending on where you live, a qualified therapist might be difficult to find). Flexibility is another appealing aspect of self-help—your loved one does all the work on his own when and where he wants to. But at the same time, it can be difficult to achieve long-lasting success with this less restrictive approach. That's because doing ERP is hard work, and no matter how good the self-help material is, it can't replace the coaching, support, and supervision given by a professional. Still, using these materials can help your relative understand OCD and prepare for working with a clinician. With this in mind, consider the following:

- Self-help is not recommended as a stand-alone treatment for OCD, but your loved one can use these resources along with a therapist.

- The majority of self-help resources are for adults, although some books are available for children and families.

- Although they are based on the principles of ERP, most self-help programs have not been rigorously researched.

- These resources are best used as a way to introduce your loved one to therapy.

- A list of self-help books for OCD can be found at *https://iocdf.org/books*.

- A list (and review) of smartphone applications for OCD can be found at *https://iocdf.org/ocd-apps*.

- The OCD Challenge website hosts a free online treatment program at *www.ocdchallenge.com*.

Standard Individual ERP

The most common way that adults and children with OCD receive ERP is by working individually with a trained clinician (later in this chapter I'll help you find a qualified provider for your loved one). Typically, treatment consists of weekly appointments and begins with a few sessions of assessment and treatment planning followed by 10–15 sessions of practice doing ERP. During the session, exposure practice is supervised by the therapist; if you're the parent of a younger child, you might be asked to attend some of these sessions. Your relative will also be asked to complete daily exposure practices and to work on resisting rituals (response prevention) between sessions (as "homework"). This is the approach that's been tested most frequently in clinical studies, and it can be extremely effective. That said, here are some things to keep in mind when thinking about this form of therapy for your loved one:

- Your loved one will have to be open and honest with her therapist about her OCD symptoms.

- She'll have to work hard at practicing exposure therapy on her own between sessions to achieve long-lasting results.

- She'll also have to be able to limit her ritualizing for treatment to be effective.

- Severe depression can interfere with the effectiveness of this approach.

- For many people with OCD, working with a therapist online (using "teletherapy") can be just as effective as face-to-face therapy and may sometimes have *advantages* over doing ERP in the office.

Couple-Based ERP for Adults

Because OCD symptoms and relationship functioning are interconnected (as you read in Chapter 3), clinicians with expertise in both couple therapy and OCD may involve a spouse or partner in ERP to directly address the ways in which the relationship impacts OCD and vice versa. Couple-based treatment involves both partners coming to all sessions and begins with an assessment of OCD symptoms, accommodation patterns, and other ways OCD interferes with the relationship. The couple is then educated about OCD, anxiety, and how ERP works. This helps increase patience and hopefulness and reduce misunderstanding and criticism. Couples are then taught how to use the types of communication skills you learned about in Chapter 7 (as well as other skills) to practice ERP successfully as a team. To the extent that accommodation is present, treatment also targets these interaction patterns. Issues not necessarily related to OCD—such as arguments about finances or child care—may also be addressed since they increase stress, interfere with teamwork, and exacerbate OCD. Here are a few additional considerations:

- Couple therapy will be helpful to the extent that you and your partner with OCD are able to work together as a team. Too much hostility and criticism will interfere, and your partner will be better off in individual therapy.

- You'll need to be optimistic and refrain from judging your partner or spouse. You'll both be assuming responsibility for progress.

- You'll need to be able to be assertive and sometimes push your partner to face her fears (in a supportive, empathic way), even though she's feeling uncomfortable.

Family–Based ERP for Children

Similar to couple therapy for adults, some ERP programs for children include parents. Within such a treatment, parents learn about OCD, the harmlessness of anxiety, and how to work with or coach their child through exposure practices and accommodation reduction in the same ways you've learned about in this book. Family-based treatment also addresses communication skills, such as how to talk about feelings and how to solve problems. Finally, parents are taught to use their leverage (as opposed to having arguments and power struggles) to shape their child's behavior with rewards and punishment and keep the child engaged in treatment. Here are some considerations it's important to keep in mind:

- Family therapy is especially helpful if your child is younger.

- It's also recommended if your child has previously had difficulty with exposure therapy. You'll learn to provide supervision and rewards to keep treatment moving forward.

- Consider this approach if your child has trouble explaining herself and her OCD. You'll be able to help with interpreting her experiences for the therapist.

- You'll need to be optimistic and supportive for family-based ERP to be successful.

Group Treatment

Studies show that ERP offered in a group setting can be as effective as individual treatment for adults and adolescents with OCD. An advantage of group therapy is that it provides built-in social support, so if your loved one feels isolated, she'll see that others face similar challenges. Other group members may also have hints, tips, and novel ways of encouraging your relative to work hard at managing obsessions and compulsions. There's something about the shared experience of tackling OCD symptoms that can be very powerful. Group therapists also work hard to foster a comfortable environment for people to share their experiences with OCD symptoms, some of which can be embarrassing. Some additional considerations are as follows:

- If your family member is afraid of speaking up in public, it can be tempting to sit back and not participate in the group, which will reduce its effectiveness.

- As with individual ERP, group therapy also requires hard work between sessions. There will be homework assignments for your relative to complete.

- Because everyone's OCD symptoms are a little different, there might not be other group members with the same sorts of obsessions and compulsions.

Intensive Outpatient Treatment

A handful of OCD specialty clinics offer intensive outpatient ERP, involving anywhere from 3 to 5 weeks of daily (Monday–Friday) treatment sessions, as opposed to weekly sessions. The main advantage of this approach, which is recommended when standard outpatient individual or group therapy hasn't been successful (or is not available), is the daily therapist contact, which helps prevent lapses between sessions. The main disadvantages include the scheduling demands and the fact that your relative might have to travel to enroll in one of these programs (or perhaps complete it online). A number of factors should guide recommendations regarding the treatment schedule. Here are some additional considerations:

- If your relative often misses weekly treatment sessions, an intensive approach might be beneficial.

- If she tries to bargain over exposure instructions or has difficulty refraining from rituals, an intensive treatment program might be worth looking into.

- It might be helpful for you to attend intensive treatment along with your loved one—even if she's an adult—so you can learn helpful ways to assist with treatment.

- The IOCDF keeps a listing of intensive treatment programs at *https:// iocdf.org/clinics.*

Day, Partial Hospitalization, and Residential Programs

The most concentrated and thorough approaches are available through day treatment, partial hospitalization, and residential (inpatient, hospitalization) programs that specialize in OCD. Here your family member (adult or child) will be admitted to a center that's specially equipped to provide ERP—usually along with other forms of treatment. Day treatment or partial hospitalization involves at least 8 hours of programming and is for people who do not require 24-hour care or supervision. Residential treatment involves being admitted to a facility that can provide an even more intensive level of care. Take note that these specialty programs are very different from your local hospital or typical state-run psychiatric facility which likely do not specialize in OCD and do not have experts trained to provide ERP. OCD specialty programs, however, are usually part of private facilities and are the best option for severe OCD that has not responded to medication or outpatient ERP. Length of stay at such programs may vary from a few weeks to a month or more. Additional considerations include the following:

- Specialized residential OCD programs provide constant supervision for your family member, including help with implementing ERP.

- The costs can be high.

- These programs are often helpful if, in addition to OCD, your relative has problems with depression, eating disorders, bipolar disorder, or other serious psychiatric conditions.

- These options might mean your family member will have to take a temporary leave from work or school to get treatment.

- The range of situations available for exposure practice may be constrained by the facility's setting. For example, if your son is afraid of the bathrooms in your home, these cannot be confronted if the treatment facility is out of town. This is important to discuss with program staff before enrolling.

- Although you might be able to visit your loved one in a residential program, it's unlikely you'd be able to be involved in her treatment to a great extent.

- The IOCDF keeps a listing of day, partial, and residential treatment programs that specialize in OCD at *https://iocdf.org/clinics*.

Stepped Care

Given the variety of treatment options available, I frequently recommend what's become known as a "stepped care" approach to the treatment of OCD. In stepped care, your family member begins with the most *effective*, yet least *intensive*, treatment and only "steps up" to more intensive services as they're needed. For example, he might begin with once-weekly therapist visits and only increase the frequency of appointments (for example, to twice weekly) if it's clear that once a week is not enough. The benefit of stepped care is that it allows you and your family to get the most out of the least amount of resources. And most experts agree with this approach. In fact, in many cases, the gatekeepers of intensive treatment programs (such as residential programs) will require that your loved one undergo a course of less intensive (such as weekly outpatient) ERP before being admitted into their intensive program.

Finding a Qualified Clinician

Where to Look

As I mentioned, not all mental health providers are well trained to use the ERP techniques that are effective for OCD. So you'll likely have to shop around before you find someone qualified to help your family member. One of the best ways to locate capable therapists in your area is by asking the leaders or members of local OCD support groups. The IOCDF website (*www.iocdf.org*) provides a list of these groups (and of IOCDF-affiliated organizations), and even if the nearest one is some distance from you, they may know of good therapists in your area or those who offer treatment online.

There are also several organizations with websites that allow you to search for mental health professionals. For several reasons, I again recommend starting with the IOCDF. For one thing, this organization is highly specialized, pouring all of its resources into advocating for people with OCD and their families. Their searchable database is maintained regularly so that it stays up to date. What I also like about this site is that it allows you to search for specific qualifications, such as whether clinicians specialize in adults or children (or both), whether they have particular specialty areas (such as washing rituals or obsessions about religion), what particular treatment strategies they use (such as ERP or ACT), and a description of their background and training. Finally, this site allows you to see whether the professional has completed the IOCDF's Behavior Therapy Training Institute (BTTI). This institute is a state-of-the-art instructional and supervision experience in which the professional receives intensive in-person training in effective ERP techniques for OCD, followed by continuing consultation with one of the institute's faculty for an additional 6 months. Individuals who have completed this program are most likely to be qualified to help your loved one.

The Association for Behavioral and Cognitive Therapies (*www.abct.org*) and the Anxiety and Depression Association of America (*www.adaa.org*) also maintain lists of professionals that you can search by name or by region. You might also be able to get referral lists from your state, provincial, or regional mental health, psychological, and psychiatric associations. And if you happen to live near a major university that has a training program in psychology or a medical school with a psychiatry department, you can call or go online and find out if they have a clinic that offers ERP.

How to Check Qualifications

Whether or not you locate a therapist through these outlets, make sure the clinician is licensed to practice in your state or province. Then ask for a description of the practitioner's qualifications and treatment approach (by e-mail or phone, rather than paying for an initial session to get this information). Here are some questions to ask a potential treatment provider and the answers you should be looking for. Don't be afraid to ask these kinds of questions—it's important that you make sure your relative is getting the treatment she needs. Speaking for myself, I appreciate it when potential patients and families ask about my qualifications because it means they're invested in treatment.

Q. What kind of treatment approach do you use for OCD?

A. Behavioral or cognitive-behavioral.

ERP and ACT are good also. But anything like gestalt, psychodynamic, eclectic, psychoanalytic, interpersonal, humanistic, Rogerian, or Jungian indicates this is not the person you're looking for.

Q. Can you tell me what ERP involves? What would the therapy be like?

A. Help with facing feared situations and refraining from rituals.

If the therapist mentions biofeedback, neurofeedback, EMDR, hypnosis, relaxation, energy therapies, or thought stopping, you're not in the right place.

Q. What formal training have you had in treating OCD using ERP?

A. Graduate school with one-on-one training and supervision from an expert, or attending multiple seminars or workshops (such as the BTTI).

You want a treatment provider with formal training or someone who is in a formal training program such as an advanced graduate student in clinical psychology. Simply reading (even a lot of reading) about ERP or attending a few workshops or lectures is not enough. Take it from me: you can't learn to do good ERP in a few hours. It takes months, if not years, of training.

Q. What role can family members play in treatment? Is it OK for a partner/spouse/parent to come to treatment sessions and help between sessions?

A. The therapist should be open to including you or another family member as either an in-session or between-sessions exposure coach (I'll also show you how to coach your loved one in the next chapter). He should be willing to (at least occasionally) allow you to sit in and observe how your relative is doing exposures.

If the clinician has experience with couple or family therapy, consider this a bonus! Perhaps she can help you address communication skills and other relationship factors that may interfere with your loved one's progress with OCD.

Q. About how many people with OCD have you worked with using ERP and what kinds of results have you gotten?

A. At least 5 to 10, with at least a 50% reduction in their symptoms.

The treatment provider should sound confident that he knows how to use ERP to get good results. But be wary of a provider who *guarantees* success or a *cure*. If something sounds too good to be true, it probably is.

You may not find a professional who gets a "perfect score" on these questions, but answering most of them correctly is usually a good sign. Finally, if the clinician can't tell you how long treatment might be expected to last, you should look for someone else. CBT is a fairly time-limited process that, in outpatient settings, usually lasts for 12–20 treatment sessions. On the other hand, be skeptical of anyone promising to successfully treat OCD in fewer sessions or in a very brief amount of time.

Proven and Unproven OCD Treatments

Although there are lots of claims out there about how to treat OCD, there really is no easy fix. Research clearly shows that ERP is your relative's best bet. But that doesn't stop some treatment providers from offering questionable therapies that haven't been studied sufficiently, don't make much sense as a treatment for OCD, or have failed when they've been put to the test. It's good to be informed about which ones to steer clear of.

How Do We Know When a Treatment Works?

The gold-standard test for determining whether a treatment works is a randomized controlled trial (RCT). RCTs provide scientific proof of a treatment's effects because they include large groups of patients who are randomly assigned to treatment or control (placebo) groups. This allows researchers to conclude that the therapy itself, and not simply the hope of improvement (what's called the *placebo effect*), caused any decreases in OCD symptoms. On the other hand, personal experience (such as "hypnosis worked for me, so it must be an effective treatment for OCD") is not considered scientific evidence that a treatment works. That's because even though a remedy might seem to be working, the improvement *could* be due to other factors such as placebo effects, normal fluctuations in symptoms, empathy from a therapist, or the simultaneous use of medicines or other therapies. Therefore, treatments not tested in RCT studies must be considered questionable or unproven.

The results of many RCTs conducted over the last 50 years show that ERP produces large improvements in OCD symptoms that are substantially greater than placebo therapies. That's why we can say with confidence that this treatment is effective for OCD and that it's doing something more than simply having a placebo effect. We know, for example, that ERP reverses the particular thought and behavior patterns that contribute to OCD. Of course, the results of RCTs are based on averages, and not everyone responds equally well.

Questionable "Treatments" for OCD in Use Today

Some of the following therapies involve techniques that seem to be contrary to what we know about obsessions and compulsions. In other cases, their use is based mainly on personal experience (what's sometimes called *anecdotal evidence*). This doesn't mean these therapies *can't* work, only that at this time there are no scientific reasons to believe they'll be any more effective than a placebo for your relative. The placebo effect is a real effect, but it's likely to produce only minimal and short-lived improvements in OCD symptoms.

Thought stopping. It sounds logical enough. Your loved one snaps a rubber band on her wrist every time an obsessional thought comes to mind. Then the rubber band is replaced with yelling "STOP!" out loud, and then eventually just thinking the word *stop*. But thought stopping is based on a misunderstanding of how OCD works, so a qualified therapist wouldn't use it. In fact, trying not to think of an unwanted thought only makes the thought more intense—plus, there's no reason to try to stop obsessional thoughts since they're normal and harmless. CBT works by helping your relative lean into these kinds of thoughts.

Talk therapy (psychodynamic therapy or psychoanalysis). The goal of talk therapies is to achieve insight into the "underlying nature" of OCD by discussing prior events or your personal history. But this approach, and the Freudian theories that it's based on, are long out of date and have been refuted. So there's no good reason to expect that simply gaining insight into what caused OCD (which is usually impossible to figure out anyway) would help someone overcome it. Finally, there are no RCTs on talk therapy with OCD.

Progressive muscle relaxation. Progressive muscle relaxation (PMR) was developed in the 1920s for reducing anxiety and stress. It involves learning to relax different muscle groups, one at a time, in a certain order. PMR is often used to lower anxiety for people with medical problems such as high blood pressure and insomnia. Some therapists use it for OCD because it can lower anxiety without the need for exposure therapy. But PMR does not address the specific factors involved in OCD, so there is no good reason to expect it to work.

Energy therapies. There is a collection of therapies (such as healing touch, Thought Field Therapy, reiki, qigong, and therapeutic touch) based on the belief that energy fields flow through our bodies and cause psychological problems (like OCD) if the energy is disturbed. The therapist assesses this disturbance and works to adjust the energy field, for example by tapping specific "meridian points" on the body. But there's no scientific evidence that

OCD has anything to do with energy fields (if these even exist!) or that energy therapies are anything more than placebos. But beware: these therapies enjoy surprising popularity among some mental health clinicians.

Equine (and other animal-assisted) therapy. Also popular is animal-assisted therapy, in which your family member engages in activities with a horse or other animal (such as grooming, feeding, haltering, or leading) while the therapist observes these interactions and uses them to process thoughts and emotions. The goal is to help your relative develop skills such as accountability, responsibility, self-confidence, problem-solving skills, and self-control. Although it is pleasant and relaxing, there are no RCTs to show that animal-assisted therapy is effective for the treatment of OCD or that it even works as an adjunct to ERP.

Biofeedback and neurofeedback. Biofeedback uses real-time electronic monitoring to help a person become aware of, and control, bodily functions such as heart rate and muscle tension. For example, someone with chronic headaches can be taught to recognize tension in his shoulders, neck, and head by seeing feedback (such as different colors on a computer screen) from a sensor that monitors muscle tension. He would then practice relaxing these muscles to reduce the headaches. Biofeedback has a long history of successful use for problems in which stress and anxiety affect medical conditions, such as headaches and high blood pressure. But there are no studies looking at biofeedback for OCD.

Neurofeedback is a new variation of biofeedback in which real-time displays of brain activity are used to teach a person how to regulate her own brain functioning. During treatment sessions, "unhealthy" brain waves are identified and monitored (via a sensor placed on the scalp), and your relative is trained to produce "healthier" brain wave patterns resulting in fewer OCD symptoms. Although it is intriguing, research on neurofeedback is insufficient (and funded by companies that sell neurofeedback equipment). But more importantly, there's no scientific basis for how neurofeedback would reduce OCD symptoms. Even the idea that OCD is associated with unhealthy brain waves (and that changing brain waves would affect OCD symptoms) is not supported by any research. In the end, many experts agree that despite lots of hype, any benefits of neurofeedback are likely placebo effects and outweighed by the high cost and time-consuming nature of this therapy.

Hypnosis. There are lots of mysteries about hypnosis and how it works. On a simple level, it provides a state of deep relaxation, which some practitioners think helps to neutralize obsessional fear. But as you've read, effective treatment for OCD does not involve helping people relax, so there's no good rationale for why hypnosis would be effective. There are also no RCTs that have tested hypnosis as a treatment for OCD, and only a very few anecdotal reports.

EMDR. EMDR, which stands for eye movement desensitization and reprocessing, was developed as a treatment for PTSD. It is sometimes used for OCD because it involves procedures similar to exposure therapy: purposely thinking about distressing images and memories. But while thinking of these images, the patient moves her eyes from side to side (for example, by following the therapist's fingers back and forth), which is thought to help move the images to a more functional part of the brain (a theory that has not been supported). Although there are a few anecdotal reports and one RCT testing EMDR for OCD, the results are not encouraging and there is no information about long-term effects. Moreover, many studies indicate that any improvement is linked to the exposure-like aspects of the therapy and that the eye movements are unnecessary.

Attention training. People with OCD tend to pay more attention to threatening information than to neutral or positive information. This "attention bias" results in perceiving the world as more dangerous than it really is. So some researchers have developed a therapy that involves training people to pay more attention to positive or neutral stimuli so they get a more objective perception of reality. The training process involves repeatedly responding to words, letters, or pictures presented on a computer screen that are designed to draw attention away from negative information. Although this idea is based on scientific findings, and RCTs have been conducted with OCD patients, the effects of this therapy have generally been small, and it's not clear that any improvement in OCD symptoms lasts over time.

Transcranial magnetic stimulation (TMS). TMS is a painless, noninvasive technique that involves applying electromagnetic currents to the skull and directing them to specific parts of the brain. In a typical session, the person is awake and sitting comfortably while the operator places a magnetic coil over a part of his head. Electromagnetic pulses are applied that travel through hair, skin, muscle, and bone so they can excite the brain in ways that are thought to reduce OCD symptoms. TMS treatment requires daily sessions lasting anywhere from 5 to 40 minutes for several weeks, and people continue with their daily activities after each session.

There's lots of anecdotal evidence and some RCTs on TMS for OCD, but again, the results aren't encouraging. First, most of the research included very small numbers of patients. And even in the largest of these studies, the degree of improvement with TMS was meager, and not much better than a "sham" TMS placebo treatment. Many patients in these studies were also using other treatments at the same time, and there are few data on long-term outcomes. There are also problems with the rationale for TMS. For one thing, there's no evidence that people with OCD have abnormal brain excitability. In addition, there's no satisfactory explanation for how reducing brain excitability would reduce obsessions and compulsions. So, are OCD symptoms reduced after receiving TMS? Yes, for some people. However, we don't know how long these results last, and there's good reason to think that placebo effects play a large role. In other words, it's doubtful that TMS is worth the time and money.

Questionable Diagnostic Techniques

Finally, beware of companies, medical clinics, and even individual clinicians who say they can use genetics (through a blood sample or cheek swab), MRI images of the brain, or other biological, chemical, or medical means to confirm your loved one's diagnosis of OCD or determine what treatment is best for him. Although these assessment techniques sound high tech and compelling, there's no research showing that these kinds of pricey procedures are any more accurate or informative than a thorough face-to-face interview with a well-trained and experienced clinician who specializes in OCD. Patients and families I've seen who have used these services often tell me they feel scammed in the end. There are no genetic, brain, or other medical tests for diagnosing OCD. So please don't get taken advantage of!

What about Medications for OCD?

I've focused primarily on psychological treatments for OCD in this book, but medication also plays a role for many children and adults. In particular, the types of medications best researched for OCD are called selective serotonin reuptake inhibitors (often referred to as SSRIs). Although published studies show that SSRIs work better than a placebo, they tend to work less consistently and be less potent than ERP. Whereas any medical doctor can prescribe SSRIs, my recommendation is to work with a psychiatrist who is knowledgeable about OCD. Usually, the doses are gradually increased over weeks and months to try to find the best balance between maximizing therapeutic benefits and minimizing side effects. The SSRIs most commonly used for treating OCD include:

- Paxil (paroxetine)
- Prozac (fluoxetine)
- Luvox (fluvoxamine)
- Zoloft (sertraline)
- Anafranil (clomipramine; which is less selective toward serotonin)

It is hard to say which SSRI is *best* for OCD. The studies comparing these drugs with one another generally find no differences in effectiveness. It's even more difficult to predict how helpful a particular SSRI will be for any individual person. And your relative also needs to keep taking the medication to sustain any improvement. Even if he's been on the drug for a long time, the risk of relapse is high if it is stopped. Another drawback is that SSRIs can produce adverse effects such as constipation, diarrhea, dry mouth, sleepiness, insomnia, headaches, weight gain, and sexual difficulties.

Can combining medication and ERP give a better result than either treatment alone? The findings are mixed. Most studies show that ERP is at least as effective as, if not more effective than, medication by itself. But the combination of ERP and medication doesn't seem to be more effective than ERP alone. In other words, contrary to what you might think, medications don't supercharge ERP. On the other hand, if your relative hasn't responded after an adequate trial on an SSRI, adding ERP can lead to a better outcome.

What's Best for My Relative: ERP or Medication?

The answer to this question requires a thorough assessment and consultation with a professional who has expertise in the treatment of OCD. But here are a few points to think about:

The American Psychiatric Association has issued guidelines for the treatment of OCD (which you can find online at *https://psychiatryonline. org/pb/assets/raw/sitewide/practice_guidelines/guidelines/ocd-guide.pdf*). In summary, they recommend that ERP be the initial treatment for adults and children with OCD who are not severely depressed. An SSRI alone is only recommended for people who are not willing to do ERP or those who have previously responded well to an SSRI. Combined treatment is suggested for adults and children who have not responded to either ERP or medications alone or who are already using a medication but wish to come off the drug.

There are also trade-offs with both ERP and medication. Most important, in my opinion, is that although success with ERP requires hard work and substantial time and energy up front, this investment is likely to pay off with lasting results down the road. Medications, on the other hand, while being easy to take, have less desirable long-term outcomes, and maintaining any improvement requires staying on the drug and perhaps dealing with side effects.

Be an Informed Consumer

It's tough enough for your relative to make the decision to reach out for help, let alone figure out what type of treatment to pursue and then find the right provider. There's a lot of information to consider, and it's easy to feel overwhelmed. But you and your loved one deserve a clear understanding of who she's working with and what she can expect from treatment. Once you've located a provider you have confidence in and begin treatment, continue to ask questions during therapy. Inquiries about the speed or pace of treatment, how the therapist is assessing progress, whether a medication is needed, and whether there are adjustments in the time course expected for treatment to be complete are all worth making.

It's especially important to ask about your role in your family member's treatment—particularly if she's receiving ERP. That's because in addition to her in-session exposure practices, her therapist will want her to practice exposure and response prevention between sessions. And that's where you can be most helpful! In the next chapter, I'll teach you the skills you'll need to successfully assist your loved one at home as she works with her therapist to overcome OCD.

15

Becoming an Effective
Exposure Therapy Coach

Arriving at a place where your loved one has chosen to get professional help is a major triumph. Hopefully your relative will be working with a clinician who has experience and expertise in the treatment of OCD. If this therapist is less experienced, you or your relative might suggest using my book *Getting Over OCD: A 10-Step Workbook for Taking Back Your Life* as a guide to working through ERP. Regardless, as a parent or partner, there's space for you to be involved in treatment to one degree or another. Perhaps the therapist will want you to attend one or more appointments. Or maybe your job will be to provide support between sessions. Usually, younger children require the most hands-on supervision during treatment. If you're helping an older child, spouse, or partner, your function will be more collaborative and consultative. Your relative's therapist has the clinical judgment to decide what's in everyone's best interest. In this chapter, I'll provide a rundown of what happens during ERP treatment (in-depth descriptions are provided in *Getting Over OCD*) and tell you what you need to know to be an effective homework coach. But first, let's consider how to approach your role in your family member's treatment.

Clarifying Your Role in Treatment

If you're a parent, your primary role in the family is to provide unconditional love and support for your child with OCD, setting appropriate boundaries and limits as you prepare him for the world. Similarly, if you're the spouse or partner of someone with OCD, your purpose is to provide emotional and physical love and support and to collaborate on important decisions that affect you, your relationship, and your family. It's important not to confuse either role with that of your loved one's therapist, who must maintain a different set of boundaries and responsibilities. The therapist's job is to play a more formal role and provide help and support in an objective way. This formality and objectivity give her authority and allow her to use her best clinical judgment to be effective—which is what you're paying for!

To further stress this important point, it's worth telling you that I've worked with many parents and partners who try to take on the role of therapist with their loved one who has OCD. But this is rarely successful and it often leads to frustration. The reason is that the boundaries and responsibilities of your family role and the role of therapist are often in conflict. How could you maintain objectivity with someone you've raised since birth? How could you enforce formal professional boundaries and have authority over someone with whom you have an intimate relationship? These are some of the reasons that therapists never treat their own family members or close friends and that ethical guidelines prohibit therapists from having intimate relationships with their patients.

If you find yourself struggling to be both a relative and a therapist, step back from the more formal role and keep the role of loving and supportive parent or partner. It's perfectly appropriate for you to set boundaries and give rewards and consequences at home, but let the paid professional set rules for therapy, give homework assignments, and be the "bad guy" if things aren't going well and your loved one needs to hear difficult feedback or be persuaded to do something she's reluctant to do. As you will see in this chapter, there's plenty you can do to provide the right kind of support in your more fitting role as supportive parent or partner.

What Happens During the Treatment for OCD?

In Chapter 4, I described the techniques used in CBT for OCD—ERP being the main ingredient in effective treatment. But understanding how the treatment process unfolds session by session will help you prepare for your role in supporting your loved one's therapy. So here's a brief description of how therapy for OCD generally progresses:

Assessment. During the first few sessions, the therapist conducts a formal assessment, gets to know your loved one, and learns about all the situations, objects, thoughts, and images that trigger obsessional fear and the rituals, avoidance, and other strategies she uses to reduce anxiety. You might be asked for input as well, especially if you're the parent of a child with OCD. It's also important for the therapist to know about any ongoing accommodation patterns or relationship/family stressors that affect OCD. Your relative might be asked to keep track of obsessions and rituals between sessions to help the therapist learn even more about the frequency, intensity, and duration of these symptoms.

Education. Throughout the assessment sessions, the therapist teaches your family member about the vicious cycle of OCD (similar to what you read about in Chapter 2 of this book) and how ERP reverses this cycle. It's valuable for you to learn this information as well, especially if relationship or family factors play a role in your relative's OCD.

Treatment planning. During the next phase of treatment, the therapist and your family member work together to organize the assessment information into a treatment plan based on (1) a list of stimuli in the environment that trigger obsessional fear (the situational exposure list); (2) a list of intrusive obsessional thoughts, images, and doubts (the imaginal exposure list); and (3) a list of rituals and other anxiety reduction behaviors to be targeted in response prevention. The core of the ERP treatment plan involves your relative confronting each item on the exposure lists and working on reducing rituals on that list. The order in which your relative works on the exposure items and rituals (sometimes called a *hierarchy*) is decided collaboratively. Finally, the therapist talks with your loved one about the process of doing ERP so she's ready to get the most out of these techniques, explaining that the ERP work will begin in treatment sessions but that the bulk of it will be done as homework between sessions. Treatment planning usually takes one or two sessions, and being present at these appointments will help you help your relative once ERP begins.

Exposure. Once the planning and education process is complete (usually after three or four sessions), ERP sessions begin. After a few minutes reviewing the past week and any homework assignments, the therapist helps your relative confront the selected item(s) on her situational and imaginal exposure lists. The first exposure with each item is usually practiced during a treatment session (which might be 60–90 minutes) so it can be supervised carefully. Situational exposures might take place in the office, virtually, or on field trips to feared locations (such as a gas station or shopping mall). For imaginal exposure, your relative would practice describing the unwanted thought, image, or doubt, perhaps writing a script that can be reread during future exposures. Cognitive therapy and ACT might be introduced as needed to help your relative learn not to be afraid. Then the therapist will recommend practicing the same exposure (or similar ones) between sessions, specifying the frequency and length of these homework practices. Your loved one might be given worksheets for keeping track of progress with homework exposures. This process continues until all of the items on the exposure lists have been confronted successfully.

You may be asked to attend some or all exposure sessions with your loved one, and the therapist will give you instructions for how to provide support with homework exposures. If you have a young child, you'll probably learn how to take an active supervisory role. For an older child, you'll likely have a more hands-off, consultative role. If it's your partner or spouse with OCD, the therapist might help you work together as a couple to implement exposure practices between sessions.

Response prevention. Along with practicing exposures, your family member will be working on reducing rituals. The response prevention plan will specify whether the goal is *full* or *partial* (for example, only 10 rituals per day instead of 20) response prevention. Your family member will also be given a log to keep track of rituals he can't resist between sessions so that these can be targeted more thoroughly with the therapist. Your role will involve providing encouragement and praise for resisting urges to ritualize, as well as reducing accommodation behaviors.

Wrapping up. After your family member has completed all of the planned exposures and is able to refrain from rituals and other anxiety reduction strategies in response to obsessions, the therapist will cover strategies for responding to *lapses*—flare-ups of OCD symptoms, which are inevitable—and preventing *relapses*. Although regularly scheduled (for example, weekly) sessions might come to an end, instructions to continue with ERP practices and less frequent (or "as needed") appointments might be arranged. At this point, your relative should have the skills to be self-sufficient (or to work effectively with you) if and when obsessional fears shows up.

How to Coach Your Relative through ERP

Research shows that receiving the right kind of support during ERP dramatically increases this treatment's short- and long-term effects. As you'll learn in this section, the "right kind" of support means helping your relative *get through* exposures by leaning into anxiety, obsessional thoughts, and uncertainty, rather than providing reassurance or trying to minimize his distress. If that sounds challenging, I understand! It's no fun watching someone you love face fears without being able to step in and help. Keep in mind, though, as you learned in Chapter 6 (which might be helpful to review), anxiety, obsessions, and uncertainty are all safe and manageable experiences for your loved one. In fact, given that he's got OCD, your loved one has tons of experience dealing with this kind of distress. When you coach him through ERP, you'll simply be helping him learn to manage this distress in ways that break the cycle of OCD, rather than keep it going.

Before You Begin

The therapist will provide specific instructions for how your relative should practice each exposure task, including how long the exposure should last and how often to repeat it between sessions. So, before you begin, have a conversation with your relative to plan how the exposure will go from start to finish. Treat this as teamwork; but if he wants to take the lead, allow him to do so. In addition to working out the details of the exercise, discuss what he's afraid of. What does he think will be the most difficult part? What does he worry would happen if he does the exposure without any rituals? What will he learn from the exposure? Discuss how you will respond if he becomes very upset or wants to stop in the middle. As with anything else, the more planning you do up front, the more smoothly the exposure practice will go.

Starting the Exposure

Once your family member begins the exposure task, her goal is to remain focused on the situation, item, or thought that she's confronting. There will be anxiety, obsessions, and uncertainty, so use what you've learned about these experiences to encourage your loved one to treat them as unpleasant yet manageable. A useful metaphor is that of a schoolyard bully who's trying to frighten your relative. But instead of running away, cowering, or counterpunching, the best option is to confidently brush off his threats. You don't like that the bully is there, but you're not going to let him get under your skin! In a similar way, your relative can "stand up to" the unwanted thoughts and feelings. There should be no rituals since she's learning to break that pattern. And it's important to avoid analyzing the obsession or trying to figure out whether or not something bad will happen.

One strategy that works well is to encourage your family member to tell you what she's feeling and thinking during the exposure. Provide support by letting her know you understand how challenging it is, and at the same time let her know how proud you are that she's sticking with the task and facing her anxiety. Use the supportive statements in the box below to encourage her to persist if the going gets tough. If your loved one becomes irritable before or during an exposure exercise or criticizes your attempts to be supportive, remind her that this is hard work. And remember not to take any verbal attacks personally—they're coming from her anxiety. Don't get drawn into arguments (you might review pages 170–171 in Chapter 12 for help with avoiding arguments) and instead ask what you can do to help with the exposure. Wait to discuss any disagreements at a time when it won't interfere with the task at hand.

Eventually you'll want your adult relative to practice homework

---

Examples of Supportive Statements to Use During Exposure Practice

- Anxiety is normal and temporary. You're strong, and you can get through this!
- Anxiety feels *uncomfortable,* but it's not *dangerous.*
- Anxiety won't hurt you. It's your fight-or-flight/adrenaline system at work.
- It's worth deciding to be anxious now to get over this problem in the long run.
- Trying to control anxiety with rituals doesn't work. You need to lean into it to get better.
- You have options when it comes to these thoughts; you don't have to fight them.
- I know it's scary, but let's try to look at these obsessional thoughts as false alarms.
- Think of these unwanted thoughts as bullies. They're insecure, so let's not give in to them!
- We've got to live with some uncertainty here. Trying to get a guarantee won't work.

exposures on her own. At first, though, you'll need to be present to provide support. As time goes by, you'll phase out your company so she can learn to manage anxiety independently. Younger children, on the other hand, often require continued close supervision throughout the course of therapy.

Helping with Response Prevention

Although you can't directly "prevent" your loved one from doing rituals, you *can* encourage him to seek you out when he experiences a strong urge to ritualize and needs help resisting. In this role, give him lots of praise for asking you to help, then stay with him until the urge decreases to a manageable level. As with exposure, help your family member *get through* the anxiety and compulsive urge, rather than trying to make it go away (the coping statements in the box on the facing page can help here as well). Never use threats, physical force, or logical debate to stop your family member from ritualizing, but do use assertive communication if necessary. And remember that it's not the end of the world if your relative ends up performing the ritual, so don't let it lead to an argument—there will be other opportunities to practice resisting. But make sure the therapist is aware of any rituals (and arguments).

If you happen to observe your relative doing rituals he's not supposed to be doing, gently point this out and remind him to note it (perhaps in a diary or on a monitoring form provided by the therapist) so that it can be discussed in treatment. You could, for example, say something such as "It looked like you were having trouble just then. You should probably write that ritual down. And remember that I'd be glad to help you out next time." Acknowledge that resisting rituals is hard work and that anxiety and uncertainty are manageable experiences. If he can hold out and not give in, the distress will be temporary and he'll learn that he doesn't need to rely on rituals.

What If Anxiety Becomes Very Intense?

If and when your loved one's anxiety becomes intense during an exposure practice, it's important that you validate her discomfort and then use what you've learned to encourage her to remain in the situation so she can learn that even high levels of anxiety are safe and manageable. This means saying something like "I can see that you're feeling very fearful, which must be very intense. And I know you can get through this. Instead of fighting the anxiety so hard, ease up and give yourself a chance to see that it's a false alarm." Here are some additional strategies for when anxiety becomes intense:

- Use the bully metaphor here, too. Embolden your family member to stand her ground. Even if the bully looks and seems threatening, he's actually weak and insecure.

- A little temporary distraction is OK, such as a brief conversation about something else; but don't let your relative disengage or lose focus on the exposure task for too long.

- Play a game, watch a show, exercise, go for a walk or drive—not as a form of distraction, but to prove that anxiety doesn't have to stop your relative from doing things she likes. During the activity, remind her that she can act *despite* anxiety—even if she doesn't enjoy the activity to the fullest.

- Remind your relative that extreme anxiety is time-limited. As long as he stops fighting it, the fear will come down as time passes. Encourage him to let himself feel anxious.

Don't use intense anxiety as a reason to call off or postpone the exposure. Remember, there's no real danger here. If your loved one threatens to quit, see if you can encourage her to persevere using supportive statements like the ones in the box on page 218. For example, if your daughter says, "I can't do this, I'm too anxious," you might respond, "I can tell you're really anxious right now. Let's remind ourselves of what we talked about before we started this exposure. I know how strong you are, and I know you can get through this if you keep at it. Remember that anxiety is *uncomfortable* but not *dangerous*. This will be a great opportunity to learn that you can manage it." Physical contact, such as putting your arm around her shoulder or holding her hand, is also a very effective way to show support.

What If Your Loved One Insists on Stopping?

If your family member continues to insist on stopping the exposure despite your attempts to keep going, respect her decision and let her know you understand how difficult it is. You might say something like "OK, that was rough, but I'm glad you tried. Maybe we can try again later." Don't let any frustration you have boil over as this will provoke even more anxiety for your loved one, lead to blaming one another, and make the problem worse. Instead, put yourself in her shoes and try to understand what she's going through. Maybe everyone underestimated the difficulty of this particular exposure. Don't fall into the trap of thinking that all is lost because an exposure got derailed. But do make sure the issue is brought to the therapist's attention.

After taking some time to calm down, regroup so you can discuss what happened and plan to try the exercise again (see Linda's example on page 225). Praise your relative for agreeing to take another crack at it—after all, it's truly an act of courage. If you can pick up with the exposure right where you left off, that's great. If your loved one refuses, it's OK to modify the exercise so it's a little easier, but still challenging enough that new learning will take place. Perhaps your loved one can use the easier exposure as an intermediate step toward succeeding with the exercise you'd originally planned.

Expect setbacks from time to time and define success by how you manage them. The goal is to get through the fear, not to get rid of fear. Be sure your family member's therapist is aware of any setbacks as they'll help him understand where OCD is really digging in and where to target your efforts.

After the Exposure

After each exposure, review the experience with your loved one and discuss what he's learned from it. Has his prediction of a negative outcome changed? Has he learned that he can manage anxiety, unwanted thoughts, and uncertainty better than expected? How did his level of fear respond? How did he cope with the situation? The more you discuss what happened during the exposure, the more it solidifies his new safety learning.

Don't expect perfection and success all of the time. Recognize and reward even small gains (you might review pages 137–142 in Chapter 10 on giving rewards). Look for something you can praise even if the exercise didn't go as planned, for example, "That was a good try; you're learning how to manage with anxiety." Never belittle gradual progress. Here are some examples of helpful comments you could make following a successful exposure:

- How about that! You were convinced _____ was going to happen, but it didn't. Are you surprised?
- It seems like you're less anxious than you were in the beginning. Tell me about that.
- As you can see, anxiety is manageable, and it doesn't last forever.
- Good for you! You were very anxious, but you stuck with it. I'm proud of you.

Keep the lines of communication open by continually talking with your family member about your role in providing support. What does she like about how you're helping with ERP? What would she like you to do differently?

And understand that accomplishments might come a little at a time, so don't expect miracles or the elimination of all of your family member's obsessional anxiety and rituals. The goal is to confront the situations on the exposure list consistently so that anxiety becomes manageable.

Examples of Family–Assisted ERP

Here are descriptions of exposure practices that Eduardo, Ariel, Xavier, and Linda conducted with one of their family members serving as a coach. For full accounts of how to do exposure therapy for different types of OCD symptoms, please see *Getting Over OCD* if you need more detail.

Eduardo: Exposure to His Sister's Clothes

Eduardo's mother began by helping Eduardo identify what he specifically feared would happen when he touched his sister's shirt without doing any washing rituals. Eduardo predicted that he would become so anxious that he "couldn't stand it" and that he would feel sick almost immediately if he couldn't wash his hands or take a shower. These were the fear predictions Eduardo would test out during the ERP practice, so Eduardo's mother wrote them down.

Next, she gave Eduardo one of his sister's shirts to hold. When Eduardo asked if it was a clean or dirty shirt, his mother said that it was best if she didn't answer that question. But she also pointed out that *she'd* had no trouble handling the same clothes Eduardo would be handling. Eduardo was encouraged to hold the shirt with his whole hand, not just his fingertips, and then to touch it to his face, hair, and clothing so that he felt that every part of him was contaminated. For the next 20 minutes, Eduardo held the shirt, regularly touching it to his face, hair, and clothes. Every 5 minutes or so, his mother checked in about how Eduardo was feeling and praised him for doing a great job despite feeling anxious.

Next, Eduardo and his mother went into Eduardo's bedroom, where Eduardo touched his sister's shirt to objects in his room that he'd been avoiding when feeling contaminated, including his bed, pillow, phone, baseball caps, and his own clothes.

After 45 minutes, Eduardo and his mother decided to end the exposure because Eduardo was feeling more comfortable and said he wasn't afraid of his sister's shirt anymore. His mother gave him lots of praise for his hard work, especially the successful response prevention (no washing), and they planned to repeat the same exercise each day of the week with different pieces of his sister's clothing (pants, socks, underwear).

Ariel: Imaginal Exposure to Uncertainty about Grading Papers

Ariel and Ben began by discussing the aim of the exposure, which was for Ariel to confront her obsessional doubts about grading her students' work and refrain from checking or asking for assurances for response prevention. Since she often obsessed that such a mistake would ruin students' lives, these feared consequences were included in the imaginal exposure script that she composed. When Ben asked her what she was most afraid of, Ariel said it was not knowing whether she'd made a mistake—perhaps she'd *never* be able to know for sure if she didn't check the students' papers. So Ariel and Ben worked together to write the following script to provoke her obsessional thought and uncertainty, making sure not to include any reassuring text:

> *I graded my 9th-grade social studies students' term papers last week, and now I keep having thoughts that I made some mistakes. What if I didn't give students the grades they really deserved? What if I entered the wrong grade in my spreadsheet? My mistakes could ruin their lives. If I give a student a grade that's lower than she deserves, it could be the difference between getting into college and getting rejected. If I gave too high a grade, other teachers might think they're better students than they really are and expect too much of them. This will lead them to fail and not get into college. It would be all my fault. I really want to go back and make sure I didn't make any mistakes, but I know I can't do that. I'll always have to live with the uncertainty of whether I ruined a child's life. There's one student in particular, Dustin, that I'm most concerned about. When I was reading Dustin's paper, I remember worrying about whether I should give him an A– or a B+. I settled on a B because his paper didn't seem as good as some of the others. But I was in a bad mood that day because I'd had a fight with Ben. What if that influenced my decision about Dustin's paper? I'll never know.*

Ariel practiced by reading the script over and over several times while focusing on the uncertainty. At first her fear level spiked and she thought about ending the exposure, but Ben encouraged her to stick with it. After a while, her level of fear began to subside. Ariel remained moderately anxious, but refrained from asking Ben for assurances, which Ben praised. She was learning that feeling uncertain about the class grades was something she could tolerate. After 30 minutes, Ben suggested that Ariel take their daughter out to run an errand she needed to take care of to prove that it was possible to be productive despite feeling anxious and uncertain. Ariel agreed. Upon returning, she felt even more confident in her ability to manage uncertainty. She and Ben wrapped up by discussing the exposure. Ariel had learned that she was able to manage uncertainty about this situation without checking. Ben gave Ariel lots of praise for her resolve to get through the exposure.

Xavier: Exposure to Praying while Distracted

Xavier's bedtime prayers and Bible study were important to him, so he and his father decided to use this time to conduct an exposure. They first discussed how it would go: For exposure, Xavier would say prayers and study the Bible while his father distracted him by making noises—quietly at first, but gradually becoming louder. Xavier's response prevention task was to continue without repeating any prayers or going over what he'd studied. His main fear was that God would be upset with him for not giving these holy activities his undivided attention; and he predicted that he wouldn't be able to last for more than 3 minutes without repeating prayers or going back over what he'd studied. This was something he and his father could test out during the exposure.

So Xavier began reciting prayers while his father hummed and sang songs in the background. Xavier could feel his anxiety building, along with the urge to repeat the prayers, since he wasn't concentrating on them 100%. At first he had trouble resisting the urge, although he informed his father each time he ritualized. After a few tries, however, Xavier was able to refrain from repeating prayers. In fact, after 10 minutes, his father pointed out that Xavier had exceeded his prediction of being able to last only 3 minutes without rituals. They next repeated the exposure with Xavier studying parts of the Bible that were especially meaningful to him.

After Xavier was able to go for 15 minutes without rereading, his father suggested Xavier consider that God might be upset about what had taken place. So Xavier allowed himself to focus on the fact that he couldn't be sure what God thought of his incomplete praying and Bible study. Perhaps God was offended. This provoked distress, and Xavier asked his father to assure him that God wasn't offended. His father refrained, saying, "I don't know God's thoughts any more than you do. We've got to rely on faith." Although Xavier knew he couldn't have the answer to this question, by repeating similar exposure practices for several evenings, he learned that he was able to manage his uncertainty better than he'd thought.

Linda: Exposure to Changing Emma's Diaper

Nicholas helped with Linda's exposure to changing Emma's diaper during one of Emma's visits to their home. Linda was fearful of seeing and touching the 3-month-old baby when she was naked. The couple began by discussing Linda's fear—that pedophile thoughts would get stuck in her head and be unbearable. Nicholas listened carefully and put himself in his wife's shoes: "I know this is scary for you. It's your most challenging exposure yet. But you're ready! You can do this! And I'm here to help you get through it." They planned exactly what would happen during the exposure: Linda would put Emma on the bed, take off Emma's clothes and dirty diaper, clean her bottom, and then put on a new diaper. Nicholas would be standing nearby, and for response prevention, Linda was not allowed to ask for reassurance. She was to "just notice" any unwanted thoughts that came to mind. The goal was to change the diaper regardless of what thoughts or anxiety showed up.

Linda let Nicholas know she was feeling very anxious as she began the exposure, and Nicholas praised her for bravely facing her fear and undressing Emma. But as she started to take off the diaper, Linda said she couldn't go on. Nicholas tried more encouragement—even when Linda started crying and saying that she wasn't ready. But Linda said she needed to take a break. Nicholas persuaded Linda to instead watch *him* change Emma as a step before doing it herself. Linda agreed and was able to watch the entire changing process. Nicholas praised Linda for watching—it was not the planned exposure, but it still was more difficult than any of Linda's previous exposures. Afterward, the couple discussed what the experience was like for Linda. Linda said that just watching provoked lots of anxiety and unwanted thoughts, but she knew she had to stick it out to be successful. She then agreed to retry the planned exposure and change Emma herself later that day.

When Linda was ready to restart the exposure, she and Nicholas again discussed the procedure. Nicholas reminded Linda of how she'd previously been able to manage the intrusive thoughts and gave her lots of praise and encouragement for not giving up. Linda was determined, and she successfully changed the baby's diaper while allowing unwanted thoughts to come to mind without trying to fight them off. Afterward, she told Nicholas that the thoughts and anxiety weren't as intense as she thought they'd be. She also said that watching Nicholas change Emma earlier that day had increased her confidence that she could do it on her own. When Emma's parents came to pick up their child, Linda found herself wishing she had more time to spend with her granddaughter and she looked forward to the next visit!

Managing Common Obstacles

Here are some difficulties you might run into as you coach your relative through ERP, as well as solutions you can use to resolve them. It's never a bad idea to consult the therapist for help as well.

Continued Ritualizing

If your loved one has difficulty with response prevention and continues to do rituals, or actively tries to conceal them from you and her therapist, assertively raise your concern without becoming angry. For example, say something like "I noticed you checking the front door lock five or six times when you were about to leave the house this weekend. When we started treatment, we agreed you would ask me for help if you were having trouble resisting urges to check. What can we do so we can work together to help you get better?" If your relative responds with a renewed agreement to work more collaboratively, don't pursue the issue further.

If, however, significant infractions continue on a regular basis, make sure the therapist is aware of the situation. It might mean that treatment needs to be put on hold until your family member feels she's prepared to follow through with all the requirements. In the long run, it's wiser to postpone treatment than carry it out improperly and risk failure and disappointment.

Replacement Rituals

It's also possible your family member will find other anxiety reduction strategies to substitute for the compulsive acts he's no longer allowed to perform according to the response prevention plan. Eduardo, for example, began using hand sanitizer once he was instructed to resist washing his hands. Ariel used her phone to take pictures of the doors so she could reassure herself that they were locked without going to check them. But these "replacement rituals" are just as detrimental as the originals and therefore just as important to stop. So be on the lookout and occasionally ask if your loved one is doing anything new to relieve anxiety now that she's not allowed to ritualize.

Continued Subtle Avoidance

Perhaps your loved one is doing the required exposure without rituals, but she continues to avoid situations related to her OCD symptoms. Linda, for example, hung pictures of Emma on the wall for exposure, but then made certain not to look at them when she was walking around the house. Eduardo was able to hug his father without immediately changing his clothes, but he then avoided his bed so as not to contaminate it. These kinds of subtle avoidance behaviors reflect a reluctance to lean into anxiety, and they prevent treatment from being successful. Therefore, they should be brought to your loved one's attention and addressed, for example, "Linda, I've noticed that you look away whenever you walk by the pictures of Emma. Would it upset you to look at them?" If the answer is yes, then confronting the very situation being avoided should be added to the exposure list.

Moving Forward with Realistic Expectations

Maybe your loved one's problems with OCD recently came to light; or perhaps they've been part of your family or relationship for a long time. Either way, as you've learned in this book, it's normal to feel frustrated and impatient when OCD affects your household. It's also normal to want desperately for treatment to progress smoothly and result in complete symptom reduction. Finally, it's natural to feel disappointment and anger when things don't seem to be going in the right direction. But it's important to keep your expectations in check. Most of the ideas and techniques I've presented in this book take time, effort, and a mountain of determination to implement. And even then, your relative will remain prone to strong anxiety reactions from time to time.

What I'm trying to say is *don't expect perfection!* The fact that your child still becomes anxious in certain situations doesn't mean all is lost. And you haven't failed just because you and your spouse or partner occasionally grapple with his obsessions and compulsions. Not in the least! Never give up and never get down on yourself. After reading this book, you've got the knowledge and tools to respond in supportive ways and get things back on track (review Chapter 13 for advice on how to *keep* things on track). You know the importance of keeping your cool and (crucially) focusing on your own behavior, rather than trying to control your family member. You've also learned that you've got to take time to care for yourself so you're fresh and prepared for the challenges ahead. Take advantage of this wisdom, and you'll always be in the game.

Resources

Books

Abramowitz, Jonathan S. *Getting Over OCD: A 10-Step Workbook for Taking Back Your Life* (2nd ed.). New York: Guilford Press, 2018.

Ciarrocchi, Joseph. *The Doubting Disease: Help for Religious Obsessions and Compulsions*. Mahwah, NJ: Paulist Press, 1995.

Grayson, Jonathan. *Freedom from Obsessive–Compulsive Disorder*. New York: Berkley, 2004.

Norton, Peter J., and Martin M. Antony. *The Anti-Anxiety Program: A Workbook of Proven Strategies to Overcome Worry, Panic, and Phobias* (2nd ed.). New York: Guilford Press, 2021.

Purdon, Christine, and David A. Clark. *Overcoming Obsessive Thoughts*. Oakland, CA: New Harbinger, 2005.

Organizations That Provide Resources for People with OCD

Anxiety and Depression Association of America (ADAA)
8701 Georgia Avenue, Suite 412
Silver Spring, MD 20910
Phone: 240-485-1001
Website: *www.adaa.org*

Association for Behavioral and Cognitive Therapies (ABCT)
305 7th Avenue, 16th Floor
New York, NY 10001
Phone: 212-647-1890
Fax: 212-647-1865
E-mail: clinical.dir@abct.org
Website: *www.abct.org*

International OCD Foundation (IOCDF)
P.O. Box 961029
Boston, MA 02109
Phone: 617-973-5801
E-mail: info@iocdf.org
Website: *www.iocdf.org*

Intensive Treatment Programs

If your relative's problems with obsessions and rituals are particularly severe and she has tried CBT before but has not had much benefit, intensive outpatient treatment might be helpful. Like our program at the University of North Carolina at Chapel Hill, there are a number of clinics that offer daily (Monday through Friday) individual (one-on-one) outpatient treatment sessions for people with OCD. There are pros and cons to intensive outpatient treatment. The benefits include the fact that treatment is fairly brief, usually lasting 3–4 weeks. Most programs also have expert therapists with lots of experience. The downside is that your loved one might need to travel to get to one of these programs and may also need to put life on hold while undergoing the therapy. You can find lists of these programs at the following websites:

> International OCD Foundation: *https://iocdf.org/clinics*
>
> OCD Canada: *http://ocdcanada.org*
>
> OCD United Kingdom: *www.ocduk.org*
>
> OCD Action (also in the UK): *www.ocdaction.org.uk*
>
> OCD Ireland: *www.ocdireland.org*
>
> Mental Health Foundation of New Zealand: *www.mentalhealth.org.nz/get-help/a-z/resource/17/obsessive-compulsive-disorder*

Index

About the Author

Jonathan S. Abramowitz, PhD, is Professor of Psychology and Neuroscience, Research Professor of Psychiatry, and Director of the Anxiety and Stress Disorders Clinic at the University of North Carolina at Chapel Hill. He conducts award-winning research on OCD and other anxiety-related disorders and is the author of *Getting Over OCD, Second Edition,* and *The Stress Less Workbook*.